DET Review!

A Complete Study Guide and Practice Test Questions

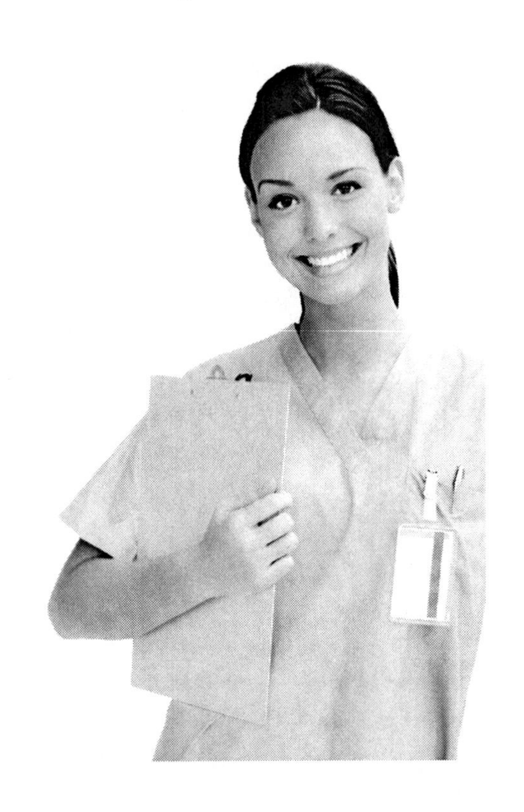

Published by

Complete TEST Preparation Inc.

We strongly recommend that students check with exam providers for up-to-date information regarding test content.

The Diagnostic Entrance Test is produced and administered by the Arnett Development Corporation, which is not affiliated with, and does not endorse this product.

978-1-77245-049-1

Version 6.5 February 2015

Published by
Complete Test Preparation
921 Foul Bay Rd.
Victoria BC Canada V8S 4H9
Visit us on the web at http://www.test-preparation.ca
Printed in the USA

Published by
Complete Test Preparation Inc.
Victoria BC Canada V8S 4H9
Visit us on the web at http://www.test-preparation.ca
Printed in the USA

About Complete Test Preparation Inc.

The Complete Test Preparation Inc. Team has been publishing high quality study materials since 2005. Thousands of students visit our websites every year, and thousands of students, teachers and parents all over the world have purchased our teaching materials, curriculum, study guides and practice tests.

Complete Test Preparation Inc. is committed to providing students with the best study materials and practice tests available on the market. Members of our team combine years of teaching experience, with experienced writers and editors, all with advanced degrees.

Team Members for this publication

Editor: Brian Stocker MA
Contributor: Dr. C. Gregory
Contributor: Dr. G. A. Stocker DDS
Contributor: D. A. Stocker M. Ed.

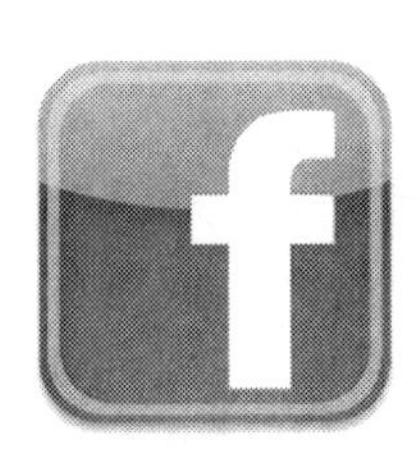

Contents

Getting Started

CONGRATULATIONS! By deciding to take the Diagnostic Entrance Test (DET) Exam, you have taken the first step toward a great future! Of course, there is no point in taking this important examination unless you intend to do your very best in order to earn the highest grade you possibly can. That means getting yourself organized and discovering the best approaches, methods and strategies to master the material. Yes, that will require real effort and dedication on your part but if you are willing to focus your energy and devote the study time necessary, before you know it you will be opening that letter of acceptance to the school of your dreams.

We know that taking on a new endeavour can be a little scary, and it is easy to feel unsure of where to begin. That's where we come in. This study guide is designed to help you improve your test-taking skills, show you a few tricks of the trade and increase both your competency and confidence.

The Diagnostic Entrance Test Exam

The DET exam is composed of modules and not all schools use all of the modules. It is therefore very important that you find out what modules your school will use! That way you won't waste valuable study time learning something that isn't on your exam!

The DET Modules are: Math, Vocabulary, Reading Comprehension, Biology, Chemistry, Physics, Basic Scientific principles and Anatomy and Physiology.

You don`t have to worry because these sections are included in this study guide. However, to maximize your study time, it is very important to check which modules your university offers before studying everything under the sun!

While we seek to make our guide as comprehensive as possible, note that like all entrance exams, the DET Exam might be adjusted at some future point. New material might be added, or content that is no longer relevant or applicable might be removed. It is always a good idea to give the materials you receive when you register to take the DET a careful review.

How this study guide is organized

This study guide is divided into four sections. The first section, Self-Assessments, which will help you recognize your areas of strength and weaknesses. This will be a boon when it comes to managing your study time most efficiently; there is not much point of focusing on material you have already got firmly under control. Instead, taking the self-assessments will show you where that time could be much better spent. In this area you will begin with a few questions to evaluate quickly your understanding of material that is likely to appear on the DET. If you do poorly in certain areas, simply work carefully through those sections in the tutorials and then try the self-assessment again.

The second section, Tutorials, offers information in each of the content areas, as well as strategies to help you master that material. The tutorials are not intended to be a complete course, but cover general principles. If you find that you do not understand the tutorials, it is recommended that you seek out additional instruction. Most Universities recommend student take introductory courses in Math, English and Science before taking the DET.

Third, we offer two sets of practice test questions, similar to those on the DET Exam. Again, we cover all modules, so make sure to check with your school!

Besides all these materials, the last three chapters give you important information on how to answer multiple choice questions, how to prepare for a test, and how to take a test.

The DET Study Plan

Now that you have made the decision to take the DET, it is time to get started. Before you do another thing, you will need to figure out a plan of attack. The very best study tip is to start early! The longer the time period you devote to regular study practice, the more likely you will be to retain the material and be able to access it quickly. If you thought that 1x20 is the same as 2x10, guess what? It really is not, when it comes to study time. Reviewing material for just an hour per day over the course of 20 days is far better than studying for two hours a day for only 10 days. The more often you revisit a particular piece of information, the better you will know it. Not only will your grasp and understanding be better, but your ability to reach into your brain and quickly and efficiently pull out the tidbit you need, will be greatly enhanced as well.

The great Chinese scholar and philosopher Confucius believed that true knowledge could be defined as knowing both what you know and what you do not know. The first step in preparing for the DET Exam is to assess your strengths and weaknesses. You may already have an idea of what you know and what you do not know, but evaluating yourself using our Self- Assessment modules for each of the three areas, Math, English and Reading Comprehension, will clarify the details.

Making a Study Schedule

To make your study time most productive you will need to develop a study plan. The purpose of the plan is to organize all the bits of pieces of information in such a way that you will not feel overwhelmed. Rome was not built in a day, and learning everything you will need to know to pass the DET Exam is going to take time, too. Arranging the material you need to learn into manageable chunks is the best way to go. Each study session should make you feel as though you have succeeded in accomplishing your goal, and your goal is simply to learn what you planned to learn during that particular session. Try to organize the content in such a way that each study session builds on previous ones. That way, you will retain the information, be better able to access it, and review the previous bits and pieces at the same time.

Self-assessment

The Best Study Tip! The very best study tip is to start early! The longer you study regularly, the more you will retain and 'learn' the material. Studying for 1 hour per day for 20 days is far better than studying for 2 hours for 10 days.

What don't you know?

The first step is to assess your strengths and weaknesses. You may already have an idea of where your weaknesses are, or you can take our Self-assessment modules for each of the areas, Math, English, Science and Reading Comprehension.

Exam Component	Rate from 1 to 5
Reading Comprehension	
Paragraph & Passage Comprehension	
Drawing inferences & conclusions	
English Grammar	
Vocabulary	
Math Fractions	
Decimals	
Percent	
Science	
Anatomy and Physiology	
Biology	
Chemistry	

Making a Study Schedule

The key to making a study plan is to divide the material you need to learn into manageable size and learn it, while at the same time reviewing the material that you already know.

Using the table above, any scores of 3 or below, you need to spend time learning, going over and practicing this subject area. A score of 4 means you need to review the material, but you don't have to spend time re-learning. A score of 5 and you are OK with just an occasional review before the exam.

A score of 0 or 1 means you really need to work on this area and should allocate the most time and the highest priority. Some students prefer a 5-day plan and others a 10-day plan. It also depends on how much time you have until the exam.

Here is an example of a 5-day plan based on an example from the table above:

Fractions: 1 Study 1 hour everyday – review on last day
Biology: 3 Study 1 hour for 2 days then ½ hour a day, then review
Vocabulary: 4 Review every second day
Word Problems: 2 Study 1 hour on the first day – then ½ hour everyday
Reading Comprehension: 5 Review for ½ hour every other day
Algebra: 5 Review for ½ hour every other day
Chemistry: 5 very confident – review a few times.

Using this example, Chemistry and Grammar are good, and only need occasional review. Biology is also good and needs 'some' review. Decimals need a bit of work, Word Problems need a lot of work and Fractions are very weak and need the majority of time. Based on this, here is a sample study plan:

Day	Subject	Time
Monday		
Study	Fractions	1 hour
Study	Word Problems	1 hour
	½ hour break	
Study	Biology	1 hour
Review	Chemistry	½ hour
Tuesday		
Study	Fractions	1 hour
Study	Word Problems	½ hour
	½ hour break	
Study	Decimals	½ hour
Review	Vocabulary	½ hour
Review	Grammar	½ hour
Wednesday		
Study	Fractions	1 hour
Study	Word Problems	½ hour
	½ hour break	
Study	Biology	½ hour
Review	Chemistry	½ hour
Thursday		
Study	Fractions	½ hour
Study	Word Problems	½ hour
Review	Biology	½ hour
	½ hour break	
Review	Grammar	½ hour
Review	Vocabulary	½ hour
Friday		
Review	Fractions	½ hour
Review	Word Problems	½ hour
Review	Biology	½ hour
	½ hour break	
Review	Vocabulary	½ hour
Review	Grammar	½ hour

Reading Comprehension Self-Assessment

THIS SECTION CONTAINS A SELF-ASSESSMENT AND READING COMPREHENSION TUTORIALS. The Tutorials are designed to familiarize general principles and the Self-Assessment contains general questions similar to the questions likely to be on the DET exam, but are not intended to be identical to the exam questions. Many Universities recommend that students take an introductory courses before taking the DET Exam. The tutorials are not designed to be a complete course, and it is assumed that students have some familiarity with reading comprehension. If you do not understand parts of the tutorial, or find the tutorial difficult, it is recommended that you seek out additional instruction.

The purpose of the self-assessment is:

- Identify your strengths and weaknesses.
- Develop your personalized study plan (above)
- Get accustomed to the DET format
- Extra practice – the self-assessments are almost a full 3rd practice test!

Since this is a Self-assessment, and depending on how confident you are with Reading Comprehension, timing is optional. The DET has 47 reading comprehension questions, to be answered in 60 minutes. Note that some schools do not have a time limit. The self-assessment has 10 questions, so allow about 13 minutes to complete this assessment.

The questions below are not the same as you will find on the DET - that would be too easy! And nobody knows what the questions will be and they change all the time. Below are general Reading Comprehension questions that cover the same areas as the DET. So the format and exact wording of the questions may differ slightly, and change from year to year, if you can answer the questions below, you will have no problem with the Reading Comprehension section of the DET.

The self-assessment is designed to give you a baseline score in the different areas covered. Here is a brief outline of how your score on the self-assessment relates to your understanding of the material.

75% - 100%	Excellent – you have mastered the content
50 – 75%	Good. You have a working knowledge. Even though you can just pass this section, you may want to review the Tutorials and do some extra practice to see if you can improve your mark.
25% - 50%	Below Average. You do not understand the reading comprehension problems. Review the tutorials, and retake this quiz again in a few days, before proceeding to the rest of the practice test questions.
Less than 25%	Poor. You have a very limited understanding of the reading comprehension problems. Please review the Tutorials, and retake this quiz again in a few days, before proceeding to the rest of the practice test questions.

After taking the Self-Assessment, use the table above to assess your understanding. If you scored low, read through the Tutorial, Help with Reading Comprehension.

Self-Assessment Answer Sheet

1. (A) (B) (C) (D)
2. (A) (B) (C) (D)
3. (A) (B) (C) (D)
4. (A) (B) (C) (D)
5. (A) (B) (C) (D)
6. (A) (B) (C) (D)
7. (A) (B) (C) (D)
8. (A) (B) (C) (D)
9. (A) (B) (C) (D)
10. (A) (B) (C) (D)
11. (A) (B) (C) (D)
12. (A) (B) (C) (D)
13. (A) (B) (C) (D)
14. (A) (B) (C) (D)

Directions: The following questions are based on several reading passages. Each passage is followed by a series of questions. Read each passage carefully, and then answer the questions based on it. You may reread the passage as often as you wish. When you have finished answering the questions based on one passage, go right onto the next passage. Choose the best answer based on the information given and implied.

Questions 1 – 4 refer to the following passage.

Passage 1 - The Immune System

An immune system is a system of biological structures and processes that protects against disease by identifying and killing pathogens and other threats. The immune system can detect a wide variety of agents, from viruses to parasitic worms, and distinguish them from the organism's own healthy cells and tissues. Detection is complicated as pathogens evolve rapidly to avoid the immune system defences, and successfully infect their hosts.

The human immune system consists of many types of proteins, cells, organs, and tissues, which interact in an elaborate and dynamic network. As part of this more complex immune response, the human immune system adapts over time to recognize specific pathogens more efficiently. This adaptation process is called "adaptive immunity" or "acquired immunity" and creates immunological memory. Immunological memory created from a primary response to a specific pathogen, provides an enhanced response to future encounters with that same pathogen. This process of acquired immunity is the basis of vaccination. [1]

1. What can we infer from the first paragraph in this passage?

a. When a person's body fights off the flu, this is the immune system in action

b. When a person's immune system functions correctly, they avoid all sicknesses and injuries

c. When a person's immune system is weak, a person will likely get a terminal disease

d. When a person's body fights off a cold, this is the circulatory system in action

2. The immune system's primary function is to:

a. Strengthen the bones

b. Protect against disease

c. Improve respiration

d. Improve circulation

3. Based on the passage, what can we say about evolution's role in the immune system?

a. Evolution of the immune system is an important factor in the immune system's efficiency

b. Evolution causes a person to die, thus killing the pathogen

c. Evolution plays no known role in immunity

d. The least evolved earth species have better immunity

4. Which sentence below, taken from the passage, tell us the main idea of the passage?

a. The human immune system consists of many types of proteins, cells, organs, and tissues, which interact in an elaborate and dynamic network.

b. An immune system is a system of biological structures and processes that protects against disease by identifying and killing pathogens and other threats.

c. The immune system can detect a wide variety of agents, from viruses to parasitic worms, and distinguish them from the organism's own healthy cells and tissues.

d. None of these express the main idea.

Questions 5 – 8 refer to the following passage.

Passage 2 - White Blood Cells

White blood cells (WBCs), or leukocytes (also spelled "leucocytes"), are cells of the immune system that defend the body against both infectious disease and foreign material. Five different and diverse types of leukocytes exist, but they are all produced and derived from a powerful cell in the bone marrow known as a hematopoietic stem cell. Leukocytes are found throughout the body, including the blood and lymphatic system.

The number of WBCs in the blood is often an indicator of disease. There are normally between 4×10^9 and 1.1×10^{10} white blood cells in a liter of blood, making up about 1% of blood in a healthy adult. The physical properties of white blood cells, such as volume, conductivity, and granularity, changes due to the presence of immature cells, or malignant cells.

The name white blood cell derives from the fact that after processing a blood sample in a centrifuge, the white cells are typically a thin, white layer of nucleated cells. The scientific term leukocyte directly reflects this description, derived from Greek leukos (white), and kytos (cell). [2]

5. What can we infer from the first paragraph in this selection?

a. Red blood cells are not as important as white blood cells.
b. White blood cells are the culprits in most infectious diseases.
c. White blood cells are essential to fight off infectious diseases.
d. Red blood cells are essential to fight off infectious diseases.

6. What can we say about the number of white blood cells in a liter of blood?

a. They make up about 1% of a healthy adult's blood.
b. There are 10^{10} WBCs in a healthy adult's blood.
c. The number varies according to age.
d. They are a thin white layer of nucleated cells.

7. What is a more scientific term for "white blood cell?"

a. Red blood cell
b. Anthrocyte
c. Leukocyte
d. Leukemia

8. Can the number of leukocytes indicate cancer?

a. Yes, the white blood cell count can indicate disease.
b. No, the white blood cell count is not a reliable indicator.
c. Disease may indicate a high white blood cell count.
d. None of the choices are correct.

Questions 9 - 12 refer to the following passage.

Keeping Tropical Fish

Keeping tropical fish as home or in your office used to be very popular. Today interest has declined, but it remains as rewarding and relaxing a hobby as ever. Ask any tropical fish hobbyist, and you will hear how soothing and relaxing watching colorful fish live their lives in the aquarium. If you are considering keeping tropical fish as pets, here is a list of the basic equipment you will need.

A filter is essential for keeping your aquarium clean and your fish alive and healthy. There are different types and sizes of filters and the right size for you depends on the size of the aquarium and the level of stocking. Generally, you need a filter with a 3 to 5 times turn over rate per hour. This means that the water in the tank should go through the filter about 3 to 5 times per hour.

Most tropical fish do well in water temperatures ranging between 24 C and 26 C, though each has its own ideal water temperature. A heater with a thermostat is necessary to regulate the water temperature. Some heaters are submersible and others are not, so check carefully before you buy.

Lights are also necessary, and come in a large variety of types, strengths and sizes. A light source is necessary for plants in the tank to photosynthesize and give the tank a more attractive appearance. Even if you plan to use plastic plants, the fish still require light, although here you can use a lower strength light source.

A hood is necessary to keep dust, dirt and unwanted materials out of the tank. In some cases the hood can also help prevent evaporation. Another requirement is aquarium gravel. This will help improve the aesthetics of the aquarium and is necessary if you plan to have real plants.

9. What is the general tone of this article?

a. Formal
b. Informal
c. Technical
d. Opinion

10. Which of the following can not be inferred?

a. Gravel is good for aquarium plants.
b. Fewer people have aquariums in their office than at home.
c. The larger the tank, the larger the filter required.
d. None of the above.

11. What evidence does the author provide to support their claim that aquarium lights are necessary?

a. Plants require light.
b. Fish and plants require light.
c. The author does not provide evidence for this statement.
d. Aquarium lights make the aquarium more attractive.

12. Which of the following is an opinion?

a. Filter with a 3 to 5 times turn over rate per hour are required.

b. Aquarium gravel improves the aesthetics of the aquarium.

c. An aquarium hood keeps dust, dirt and unwanted materials out of the tank.

d. Each type of tropical fish has its own ideal water temperature.

Questions 13 - 14 refer to the following passage.

Vice President Johnson, Mr. Speaker, Mr. Chief Justice, President Eisenhower, Vice President Nixon, President Truman, reverend clergy, fellow citizens:

We observe today not a victory of party, but a celebration of freedom -- symbolizing an end, as well as a beginning -- signifying renewal, as well as change. For I have sworn before you and Almighty God the same solemn oath our forebears prescribed nearly a century and three-quarters ago.

The world is very different now. For man holds in his mortal hands the power to abolish all forms of human poverty and all forms of human life. And yet the same revolutionary beliefs for which our forebears fought are still at issue around the globe -- the belief that the rights of man come not from the generosity of the state, but from the hand of God.

We dare not forget today that we are the heirs of that first revolution. Let the word go forth from this time and place, to friend and foe alike, that the torch has been passed to a new generation of Americans -- born in this century, tempered by war, disciplined by a hard and bitter peace, proud of our ancient heritage, and unwilling to witness or permit the slow undoing of those human rights to which this nation has always been committed, and to which we are committed today at home and around the world.

Let every nation know, whether it wishes us well or ill, that we shall pay any price, bear any burden, meet any hardship, support any friend, oppose any foe, to assure the survival and the success of liberty.

This much we pledge -- and more.

John F. Kennedy Inaugural Address delivered 20 January 1961

13. What is the tone of this speech?

a. Triumphant

b. Optimistic

c. Threatening

d. Gloating

14. Which of the following is an opinion?

a. The world is very different now.

b. For man holds in his mortal hands the power to abolish all forms of human poverty and all forms of human life.

c. We dare not forget today that we are the heirs of that first revolution

d. For I have sworn before you and Almighty God the same solemn oath our forebears prescribed nearly a century and three-quarters ago.

Reading Self-Assessment Answer Key

1. A

The passage does not mention the flu specifically, however we know the flu is a pathogen (A bacterium, virus, or other microorganism that can cause disease). Therefore, we can infer, when a person's body fights off the flu, this is the immune system in action.

2. B

The immune system's primary function is to protect against disease.

3. A

The passage refers to evolution of the immune system being important for efficiency. In paragraph three, there is a discussion of adaptive and acquired immunity, where the immune system "remembers" pathogens. We can conclude, evolution of the immune system is an important factor in the immune system's efficiency.

4. B

The sentence that expresses the main idea of the passage is, "An immune system is a system of biological structures and processes that protects against disease by identifying and killing pathogens and other threats."

5. C

We can infer white blood cells are essential to fight off infectious diseases, from the passage, "cells of the immune system that defend the body against both infectious disease and foreign material."

6. A

We can say the number of white blood cells in a liter of blood make up about 1% of a healthy adult's blood. This is a fact-based question that is easy and fast to answer. The question asks about a percentage. You can quickly and easily scan the passage for the percent sign, or the word percent and find the answer.

7. C

A more scientific term for "white blood cell" is leukocyte, from the first paragraph, first sentence of the passage.

8. A

The white blood cell count can indicate disease (cancer). We know this from the last sentence of paragraph two, "The physical properties of white blood cells, such as volume, conductivity, and granularity, changes due to the presence of immature cells, or malignant cells."

9. B

The general tone is informal.

10. B

The statement, " Fewer people have aquariums in their office than at home," **cannot** be inferred from this article.

11. C
The author does not provide evidence for this statement.

12. B
The following statement is an opinion, " Aquarium gravel improves the aesthetics of the aquarium."

13. A
This is a triumphant speech where President Kennedy is celebrating his victory.

14. C
The statement, "We dare not forget today that we are the heirs of that first revolution" is an opinion.

Help with Reading Comprehension

At first sight, reading comprehension tests look challenging especially if you are given long essays to answer only two to three questions. While reading, you might notice your attention waning, or feeling sleepy. Do not be discouraged because there are various tactics and long range strategies that make comprehending even long, boring essays easier.

Your friends before your foes. It is always best to tackle essays or passages with familiar subjects rather than those with unfamiliar ones. This approach applies the same logic as tackling easy questions before hard ones. Skip passages that do not interest you and leave them for later when you have more time.

Don't use 'special' reading techniques. This is not the time for speed-reading or anything like that – just plain ordinary reading – not too slow and not too fast.

Read through the entire passage and the questions before you do anything. Many students try reading the questions first and then looking for answers in the passage thinking this approach is more efficient. What these students do not realize is that it is often hard to navigate in unfamiliar roads. If you do not familiarize yourself with the passage first, looking for answers become not only time-consuming but also dangerous because you might miss the context of the answer you are looking for. If you read the questions first you will only confuse yourself and lose valuable time.

Familiarize yourself with reading comprehension questions. If you are familiar with the common types of reading comprehension questions, you are able to take note of important parts of the passage, saving time. There are six major kinds of reading comprehension questions.

- **Main Idea**- Questions that ask for the central thought or significance of the passage.

- **Specific Details** - Questions that asks for explicitly stated ideas.

- **Drawing Inferences** - Questions that ask for a statement's intended meaning.

- **Tone or Attitude** - Questions that test your ability to sense the emotional state of the author.

- **Context Meaning** – Questions that ask for the meaning of a word depending on the context.

- **Technique** – Questions that ask for the method of organization or the writing style of the author.

Read. Read. Read. The best preparation for reading comprehension tests is always to read, read and read. If you are not used to reading lengthy passages, you will probably lose concentration. Increase your attention span by making a habit out of reading.

Reading Comprehension tests become less daunting when you have trained yourself to read and understand fast. Always remember that it is easier to understand passages you are interested in. Do not read through passages hastily. Make mental notes of ideas that you think might be asked.

Reading Comprehension Strategy

When facing the reading comprehension section of a standardized test, you need a strategy to be successful. You want to keep several steps in mind:

- First, make a note of the time and the number of sections. Time your work accordingly. Typically, four to five minutes per section is sufficient. Second, read the directions for each selection thoroughly before beginning (and listen well to any additional verbal instructions, as they will often clarify obscure or confusing written guidelines). You must know exactly how to do what you're about to do!

- Now you're ready to begin reading the selection. Read the passage carefully, noting significant characters or events on a scratch sheet of paper or underlining on the test sheet. Many students find making a basic list in the margins helpful. Quickly jot down or underline one-word summaries of characters, notable happenings, numbers, or key ideas. This will help you better retain information and focus wandering thoughts. Remember, however, that your main goal in doing this is to find the information that answers the questions. Even if you find the passage interesting, remember your goal and work fast but stay on track.

- Now read the question and all the choices. Now you have read the passage, have a general idea of the main ideas, and have marked the important points. Read the question and all the choices. Never choose an answer without reading them all! Questions are often designed to confuse – stay focussed and clear. Usually the answer choices will focus on one or two facts or inferences from the passage. Keep these clear in your mind.

- Search for the answer. With a very general idea of what the different choices are, go back to the passage and scan for the relevant information. Watch for big words, unusual or unique words. These make your job easier as you can scan the text for the particular word.

- Mark the Answer. Now you have the key information the question is looking for. Go back to the question, quickly scan the choices and mark the correct one.

Understand and practice the different types of standardized reading comprehension tests. See the list above for the different types. Typically, there will be several questions dealing with facts from the selection, a couple more inference questions dealing with logical consequences of those facts, and periodically an application-oriented question surfaces to force you to make connections with what you already know. Some students prefer to answer the questions as listed, and feel classifying the question and then ordering is wasting precious time. Other students prefer to answer the different types of questions in order of how easy or difficult they are. The choice is yours and do whatever works for you. If you want to try answering in order of difficulty, here is a recommended order, answer fact questions first; they're easily found within the passage. Tackle inference problems next, after re-reading the question(s) as many times as you need to. Application or 'best guess' questions usually take the longest, so save them for last.

Use the practice tests to try out both ways of answering and see what works for you.

For more help with reading comprehension, see www.Multiple-Choice.ca .

Main Idea, Topic and Supporting Details

Identifying the main idea, topic and supporting details in a passage can feel like an overwhelming task. The passages used for standardized tests can be boring and seem difficult. Test writers don't use interesting passages or ones that talk about things most people are familiar with. Despite these obstacles, all passages and paragraphs will have the information you need to answer the questions.

The topic of a passage or paragraph is its subject. It's the general idea and can be summed up in a word or short phrase. On some standardized tests, there is a short description of the passage if it's taken from a longer work. Make sure you read the description as it might state the topic of the passage. If not, read the passage and ask yourself, "Who or what is this about?" For example:

> Over the years, school uniforms have been hotly debated. Arguments are made that students have the right to show individuality and express themselves by choosing their own clothes. However, this brings up social and academic issues. Some kids cannot afford to wear the clothes they like and might be bullied by the "better dressed" students. With attention drawn to clothes and the individual, students will lose focus on class work and the reason they are in school. School uniforms should be mandatory.

Ask: What is this paragraph about?
Topic: school uniforms

Once you have the topic, it's easier to find the main idea. The main idea is a specific statement telling what the writer wants you to know about the topic. Writers usually state the main idea as a thesis statement. If you're looking for the main idea of a single paragraph, the main idea is called the topic sentence and will probably be the first or last sentence. If you're looking for the main idea of an entire passage, look for the thesis statement in either the first or last paragraph. The main idea is usually restated in the conclusion. To find the main idea of a passage or paragraph, follow these steps:

1. Find the topic.

2. Ask yourself, "What point is the author trying to make about the topic?"

3. Create your own sentence summarizing the author's point.
4. Look in the text for the sentence closest in meaning to yours.

Look at the example paragraph again. It's already established that the topic of the paragraph is school uniforms. What is the main idea/topic sentence?

Ask: "What point is the author trying to make about school uniforms?"

Summary: Students should wear school uniforms.

Topic sentence: School uniforms should be mandatory.
Main Idea: School uniforms should be mandatory.

Each paragraph offers supporting details to explain the main idea. The details could be facts or reasons, but they will always answer a question about the main idea. What? Where? Why? When? How? How much/many? Look at the example paragraph again. You'll notice that more than one sentence answers a question about the main idea. These are the supporting details.

Main Idea: School uniforms should be mandatory.

Ask: Why?

> *Some kids cannot afford to wear clothes they like and could be bullied by the "better dressed" kids.
> **Supporting Detail**
>
> *With attention drawn to clothes and the individual, Students will lose focus on class work and the reason they are in school. **Supporting Detail**

What if the author doesn't state the main idea in a topic sentence? The passage will have an implied main idea. It's not as difficult to find as it might seem. Paragraphs are always organized around ideas. To find an implied main idea, you need to know the topic and then find the relationship between the supporting details. Ask yourself, "What is the point the author is making about the relationship between the details?"

> Cocoa is what makes chocolate good for you. Chocolate comes in many varieties. These delectable flavors include milk chocolate, dark chocolate, semi-sweet, and white chocolate.

Ask: What is this paragraph about?
Topic: Chocolate

Ask: What? Where? Why? When? How? How much/many?

Supporting details: Chocolate is good for you because it is made of cocoa, Chocolate is delicious, Chocolate comes in different delicious flavors

Ask: What is the relationship between the details and what is the author's point?

Main Idea: Chocolate is good because it is healthy and it tastes good.

Testing Tips for Main Idea Questions

1. **Skim the questions** – not the answer options - before reading the passage.

2. **Questions about main idea might use the words "theme," "generalization," or "purpose."**

3. **Save questions about the main idea for last.** On standardized tests like the SAT, the answers to the rest of the questions can be found in order in the passage.

3. **Underline topic sentences in the passage.** Most tests allow you to write in your testing booklet.

4. **Answer the question in your own words before looking at the answer options.** Then match your answer with an answer option.

5. **Cross out incorrect options immediately to prevent confusion.**

6. **If two of the options mean the same thing but use different words, they are BOTH incorrect.**

7. **If a question asks about the whole passage, cross out the options that apply to only part of it.**

8. **If only part of the information is correct, that option is incorrect.**

9. **An option that is too broad is incorrect.** All information needs to be backed up by the passage.

10. **Options with extreme wording are usually incorrect.**

Mathematics

THIS SECTION CONTAINS A SELF-ASSESSMENT AND MATH TUTORIALS. The Tutorials are designed to familiarize general principles and the Self-Assessment contains general questions similar to the math questions likely to be on the DET exam, but are not intended to be identical to the exam questions. Many Universities recommend that students take an introductory math course before taking the DET Exam. The tutorials are not designed to be a complete math course, and it is assumed that students have some familiarity with math. If you do not understand parts of the tutorial, or find the tutorial difficult, it is recommended that you seek out additional instruction.

Mathematics Self-assessment

Below is a Mathematics Self-assessment. The purpose of the self-assessment is:

- Identify your strengths and weaknesses.
- Develop your personalized study plan (above)
- Get accustomed to the DET format
- Extra practice – the self-assessments are almost a full 3rd practice test!

Since this is a Self-assessment, and depending on how confident you are with Math, timing yourself is optional. The DET includes a comprehensive Math Exam that covers decimals, whole numbers, fractions, number system conversions, percentages and basic algebra. There is generally a section where you are asked to solve medical related word problems, such as calculating dosages. There are a total of 50 questions, which must be answered in 50 minutes. The self-assessment has 50 questions, so allow 50 minutes to complete this assessment.

The questions below are not the same as you will find on the DET - that would be too easy! And nobody knows what the questions will be and they change all the time. Below are general Math questions that cover the same areas as the DET. So, while the format and exact wording of the questions may differ slightly, and change from year to year, if you can answer the questions below, you will have no problem with the Math section of the DET.

The self-assessment is designed to give you a baseline score in the different areas covered. Here is a brief outline of how your score on the self-assessment relates to your understanding of the material.

75% - 100%	Excellent – you have mastered the content
50 – 75%	Good. You have a working knowledge. Even though you can just pass this section, you may want to review the tutorials and do some extra practice to see if you can improve your mark.
25% - 50%	Below Average. You do not understand the content. Review the tutorials, and retake this quiz again in a few days, before proceeding to the rest of the practice test questions.
Less than 25%	Poor. You have a very limited understanding. Please review the Tutorials, and retake this quiz again in a few days, before proceeding to the rest of the practice test questions.

Math Self-Assessment Answer Sheet

1. (A) (B) (C) (D)
2. (A) (B) (C) (D)
3. (A) (B) (C) (D)
4. (A) (B) (C) (D)
5. (A) (B) (C) (D)
6. (A) (B) (C) (D)
7. (A) (B) (C) (D)
8. (A) (B) (C) (D)
9. (A) (B) (C) (D)
10. (A) (B) (C) (D)
11. (A) (B) (C) (D)
12. (A) (B) (C) (D)
13. (A) (B) (C) (D)
14. (A) (B) (C) (D)
15. (A) (B) (C) (D)
16. (A) (B) (C) (D)
17. (A) (B) (C) (D)
18. (A) (B) (C) (D)
19. (A) (B) (C) (D)
20. (A) (B) (C) (D)
21. (A) (B) (C) (D)
22. (A) (B) (C) (D)
23. (A) (B) (C) (D)
24. (A) (B) (C) (D)
25. (A) (B) (C) (D)
26. (A) (B) (C) (D)
27. (A) (B) (C) (D)
28. (A) (B) (C) (D)
29. (A) (B) (C) (D)
30. (A) (B) (C) (D)
31. (A) (B) (C) (D)
32. (A) (B) (C) (D)
33. (A) (B) (C) (D)
34. (A) (B) (C) (D)
35. (A) (B) (C) (D)
36. (A) (B) (C) (D)
37. (A) (B) (C) (D)
38. (A) (B) (C) (D)
39. (A) (B) (C) (D)
40. (A) (B) (C) (D)
41. (A) (B) (C) (D)
42. (A) (B) (C) (D)
43. (A) (B) (C) (D)
44. (A) (B) (C) (D)
45. (A) (B) (C) (D)
46. (A) (B) (C) (D)
47. (A) (B) (C) (D)
48. (A) (B) (C) (D)
49. (A) (B) (C) (D)
50. (A) (B) (C) (D)

Basic Math

1. 389 + 454 =

a. 853
b. 833
c. 843
d. 863

2. 9,177 + 7,204 =

a. 16,4712
b. 16,371
c. 16,381
d. 15,412

3. 2,199 + 5,832 =

a. 8,331
b. 8,041
c. 8,141
d. 8,031

4. 8,390 - 5,239 =

a. 3,261
b. 3,151
c. 3,161
d. 3,101

5. 643 - 587 =

a. 56
b. 66
c. 46
d. 55

6. 3,406 - 2,767 =

a. 629
b. 720
c. 639
d. 649

7. 149 × 7 =

a. 1032
b. 1043
c. 1059
d. 1063

8. 467 × 41 =

a. 19,147
b. 21,227
c. 23,107
d. 18,177

9. 309 × 17 =

a. 5,303
b. 4,913
c. 4,773
d. 5,253

10. 491 ÷ 9 =

a. 54 r5
b. 56 r6
c. 57 r5
d. 51 r

Decimals, Fractions and Percent

11. 15 is what percent of 200?

a. 7.5%
b. 15%
c. 20%
d. 17.50%

12. A boy has 5 red balls, 3 white balls and 2 yellow balls. What percent of the balls are yellow?

a. 2%
b. 8%
c. 20%
d. 12%

13. Add 10% of 300 to 50% of 20

a. 50%
b. 40%
c. 60%
d. 45%

14. Convert 75% to a fraction.

a. 2/100
b. 75/100
c. 3/4
d. 4/7

15. Convert 90% to a fraction

a. 1/10
b. 9/9
c. 10/100
d. 9/10

16. Multiply 3 by 25% of 40

a. 75
b. 30
c. 68
d. 35

17. What is 10% of 30 multiplied by 75% of 200?

a. 450
b. 750
c. 20
d. 45

18. Convert 0.28 to a fraction.

a. 7/25
b. 3.25
c. 8/25
d. 5/28

19. Convert 0.45 to a fraction

a. 7/20
b. 7/45
c. 9/20
d. 3/20

20. Convert 1/5 to percent.

a. 10%
b. 5%
c. 20%
d. 25%

21. Convert 4/20 to percent

a. 25%
b. 20%
c. 40%
d. 30%

22. Convert 0.55 to percent

a. 45%
b. 15%
c. 75%
d. 55%

23. Convert 0.33 to percent

a. 77%
b. 67%
c. 33%
d. 57%

24. A man buys an item for $420 and has a balance of $3000.00. How much did he have before?

a. $2,580
b. $3,420
c. $2,420
d. $342

25. Divide 9.60 by 3.2

a. 2.50
b. 3
c. 2.3
d. 6.4

26. What is the best approximate solution for 1.135 - 113.5?

a. -110
b. 100
c. -90
d. 110

Medical Dosage Problems

27. The physician orders 40 mg Depo-Medrol; 80 mg/ml is on hand. How many milliliters will you give?

a. 0.5 ml
b. 0.80 ml
c. 0.25 ml
d. 0.40 ml

28. The physician orders 750 mg Tagamet liquid; 1500 mg/tsp is on hand. How many teaspoons will you give?

a. 0.75 tsp
b. 0.5 tsp
c. 1 tsp
d. 0.55 tsp

29. The physician ordered 75 mg of Seconal; 50 mg/mL is on hand. How many mL will you give?

a. 1.25 ml
b. 1.75 ml
c. 1 ml
d. 1.5 ml

30. The physician ordered 1,500 mg Duricef; 1g/tablet is on hand. How many tablets will you give?

a. .5 tablets
b. .75 tablet
c. 1 tablet
d. 1.5 tablets

31. The physician orders 150 mg morphine sulphate; 1 g/ml is on hand. How many ml will you give?

a. 0.15 ml
b. 1.5 ml
c. 0.25 ml
d. 0.015

32. The physician ordered 10 units of regular insulin; 100 U/mL is on hand. How many milliliters will you give?

a. 1.01ml
b. 1 ml
c. 0.01 ml
d. 0.1 ml

Metric Conversion

33. Convert 10 kg. to grams.

a. 10,000 grams
b. 1,000 grams
c. 100 grams
d. 10.11 grams

34. Convert 0.55 metric tons to kilograms.

a. 55 kg.
b. 5500 kg.
c. 550 kg.
d. 505 kg.

35. Convert 2.5 liters to milliliters.

a. 1050 ml.
b. 2,500 ml.
c. 2050 ml.
d. 1500 ml.

36. Convert 210 mg. to grams.

a. 0.21 mg.
b. 2.1 g.
c. 0.21 g.
d. 2.12 g.

37. Convert 10 pounds to kilograms.

a. 4.54 kg.
b. 11.25 kg.
c. 15 kg.
d. 10.25 kg.

38. Convert 450 cm. to decameter.

a. 4500 dm.
b. 450 dm.
c. 45 dm.
d. 0.45 dm.

39. Convert 850 ml. to deciliters.

a. 8.5 dl.
b. 85 dl.
c. 8.5 ml.
d. 850 dl.

40. Convert 0.539 grams to milligrams.

a. 539 g.
b. 539 mg.
c. 53.9 mg.
d. 0.53 g.

Word Problems

41. Two trains leave a station at the same time. One has an average speed of 72km/hr. and the other 52km/hr. How far apart are they in 20 minutes?

a. 6.67 km.
b. 17.33 km.
c. 24.3 km.
d. 41.33 km.

42. The average weight of 13 students in a class of 15 (two were absent that day) is 42 kg. When the remaining two are weighed, the average became 42.7kg. If one of the remaining students weighs 48, how much does the other weigh?

a. 44.7 kg.
b. 45.6 kg.
c. 46.5 kg.
d. 47.4 kg.

43. The total expense of building a fence around a square-shaped field is $2000 at a rate of $5 per meter. What is the length of one side?

a. 40 meters.
b. 80 meters.
c. 100 meters.
d. 320 meters.

44. There were some oranges in a basket. By adding 8/5 of the total to the basket, the new total is 130. How many oranges were in the basket?

a. 60
b. 50
c. 40
d. 35

45. Two trains started at the same time from points 200 km. apart. The first train travels at 40 km/hr and the second train travels at 65 km/hr. How many minutes will it take them to cross?

a. 92 minutes.
b. 106 minutes.
c. 114 minutes.
d. 118 minutes.

46. A person earns $25,000 and pays $9,000 income tax per year. The Government increased income tax by 0.5% per month and his monthly earning was increased $11,000. How much more income tax will he pay per month?

a. $1260
b. $1050
c. $750
d. $510

47. A company gives a 12% discount to customers on the retail price, and on total purchases over $10,000, they give an additional 3% discount. A customer's total came to $13,500 (discounted price). How much did he save?

a. $2315
b. $1850
c. $2025
d. $2225

48. Brian jogged 7 times around a circular track 75 meters in diameter. How much linear distance did he cover?

a. 1250 meters
b. 1450 meters
c. 1650 meters
d. 1725 meters

49. A mother is 7 times older than her child is. In 25 years, her age will be double that of her child. How old is the mother now?

a. 25
b. 30
c. 33
d. 35

50. John purchased a jacket at a 7% discount. He had a membership that gave him an additional 2% discount. If he paid $425, what is the retail price of the jacket?

a. $448
b. $460
c. $466
d. $472

Answer Key

Basic Math

1. C
389 + 454 = 843

2. C
9,177 + 7,204 = 16,381

3. D
2,199 + 5,832 = 8,031

4. B
8,390 - 5,239 = 3,151

5. A
643 - 587 = 56

6. C
3,406 - 2,767 = 639

7. B
149 × 7 = 1043

8. A
467 × 41 = 19,147

9. D
309 × 17 = 52,53

10. A
491 ÷ 9 = 54 r5

Decimals, Percent and Fractions

11. A
15% = 15/100 X 200 = 7.5%

12. C
Total no. of balls = 10, no. of yellow balls = 2, answer = 2/10 X 100 = 20%

13. B
10% of 300 = 30 and 50% of 20 = 10 so 30 + 1- = 40.

14. C
75%= 75/100 = ¾

15. D
90% = 90/100 = 9/10

16. B
25% of 40 = 10 and 10 x 3 = 30

17. A
10% of 30 = 3 and 75% of 200 = 150, 3 X 150 = 450

18. A
0.28 = 28/100 = 7/25

19. C
0.45 = 45/100 = 9/20

20. C
1/5 X 100 = 20%

21. B
4/20 X 100 = 1/5 X 100 = 20%

22. D
0.55 X 100 = 55%

23. C
0.33 X 100 = 33%

24. B
(Amount Spent) $420 + $3000 (Balance) = $3420

25. B
9.60/3.2 = 3

26. A
1.135 -113.5 = -113.5 + 1-135 = -112.37.
Best approximate = -110

Medical Dosage Problems

27. A
Set up the formula -
Dose ordered/Dose on hand X Quantity/1 = Dosage
40 mg/80 mg X 1 ML/1 = 40/80 = 0.5 mL

28. B
Set up the formula -
Dose ordered/Dose on hand X Quantity/1 = Dosage
750 mg/1500 mg X 1 tsp/1 = 750/1500 = 0.5 tsp

29. D
75 mg/50mg X 1 mL/1 = 75/50 = 1.5 mL

30. D
1500 mg/1000 mg X 1 tab/1 = 1500/1000 = 1.5 tablets
(Convert 1 g = 1000 mg)

31. A
150 mg/1000 mg X 1ml/1 = 150/1000 = 0.15 mL (Convert 1 g = 1000 mg)

32. D
10 units/100 units X 1 ML/1 = 10/100 = 0.1 mL

Metric Conversion

33. A
1kg = 1,000 g and 10 kg = 10 x 1,000 = 10,000 g

34. C
1,000 kilograms = 1 ton, 0.55 ton = 1,000 x 0.55 = 550 kilograms

35. B
1 liter = 1,000 milliliters, 2.5 liters = 2.5 x 1,000 = 2,500 milliliters

36. C
1,000 mg = 1 g, 210 mg = 210/1,000 = 0.21 g

37. A
1 pound = 0.45 kg, 10 pounds = 4.53592, or 4.54 kg

38. D
1000 cm=1 dm, 450 cm = 1,000/450 = 0.45 dm

39. A
5.8 dl 100 ml = 1 dl., 850 ml = 850/100 = 8.5 dl.

40. B 1 g = 1,000 mg. 0.539 g = 0.539 x 1000 = 539 mg.

Word Problems

41. A
Distance traveled by 1st train in 20 minutes = (72 km/hr × 20 minutes) /60 minutes = 24 km. Distance traveled by 2nd train in 20 minutes = (52 km/hr × 20 minutes)/60 minutes = 17.33 km. Difference in distance = 24 - 17.33 = 6.67 km

42. C
Total weight of 13 students with average 42 will be = 42•13 = 546 kg.

The total weight of the remaining 2 will be found by subtracting the total weight of 13 students from the total weight of 15 students: 640.5 - 546 = 94.5 kg.

94.5 = the total weight of two students. One of these students weigh 48 kg, so;

The weight of the other will be = 94.5 – 48 = 46.5 kg

43. C
Total expense is $2000 and we are informed that $5 is spent per meter. Combining these two information, we know that the total length of the fence is 2000/5 = 400 meters.

The fence is built around a square shaped field. If one side of the square is "a," the perimeter of the square is "4a." Here, the perimeter is equal to 400 meters. So,

400 = 4a

100 = a → this means that one side of the square is equal to 100 meters

44. B
Let the number of oranges in the basket before additions = x
Then: X + 8x/5 = 130
5x + 8x = 650
X = 50

45. C
Let the time to cross be x hours. The equation will be
40x + 65x = 200
X = 1.9047 hours
X = 1.9047 X 60 = 114.28 minutes

46. D
The income tax per year is $9,000. So, the income tax per month is 9,000/12 = $750.

This person earns $25,000 per month and pays $750 income tax. We need to find the rate of the income tax:

Tax rate: 750•100/25,000 = 3%

Government increased this rate by 0.5% so it became 3.5%.

The income of the person per month is increased $11,000 so it became: $25,000 + $11,000 = $36,000.

The new monthly income tax is: 36,000•3.5/100 = $1260.

Amount of increase in tax per month is: $1260 - $750 = $510.

47. A
To calculate the balance before the 3% was taken solve the equation: 13500 = 0.97x, x = 13917.53 Then use this number to solve what the total was before the 12% discount, with the equation: 13917.53 = 0.88x, x = 15,815.37. Then subtract 13500 from this to get a savings of $2315

48. C
In one round trip he covers the distance equal to the circumference of the circular path.

Circumference/Diameter = π = 3.14159
75/X = 3.14159
75 X 3.14159 = X

Circumference of the path = X = 235.65 meters.

Distance covered 7 times around = 235.65 × 7=1650 meters.

49. D
The easiest way to solve age problems is to use a table:

	Mother	Child
Now	7x	x
25 years later	7x + 25	x + 25

Now, mother is 7 times older than her child. So, if we say that the child is x years old, mother is 7x years old. In 25 years, 25 will be added to their ages. We are told that in 25 years, mother's age will double her child's age. So,

7x + 25 = 2(x + 25) ... by solving this equation, we reach x that is the child's age:

7x + 25 = 2x + 50

7x - 2x = 50 - 25

5x = 25

x = 5

Mother is 7x years old: 7x = 7•5 = 35

50. C

Let the original price be 100x.

At the rate of 7% discount, the discount will be 100x•7/100 = 7x. So, the discounted price will be = 100x - 7x = 93x.

Over this price, at the rate of 2% additional discount, the discount will be 93x•2/100 = 1.86x. So, the additionally discounted price will be = 93x - 1.86x = 91.14x.

This is the amount which John has paid for the jacket:

91.14x = 425

x = 425 / 91.14 = 4.6631

The jacket costs 100x. So, 100x = 100•4.6631 = $466.31.

When rounded to the nearest whole number, this is equal to $466.

Metric Conversion – A Quick Tutorial

Conversion between metric and standard units can be tricky since the units of distance, volume, area and temperature can seem arbitrary when compared. Although the metric system (using SI units) is the standard system of measure in most parts of the world many countries still use at least some of their traditional units of measure. In North America those units come from the old British system.

Distance

When measuring distance the relation between metric and standard units looks like this:

0.039 in	1 millimeter	1 inch	25.4 mm
3.28 ft	1 meter	1 foot	.305 m
0.621 mi	1 kilometer	1 mile	1.61 km

Here, you can see that 1 millimeter is equal to .039 inches and 1 inch equals 25.4 millimeters.

Area

When measuring area the relation between metric and standard looks like this:

.0016 in^2	1 square millimeter	1 square inch	645.2 mm^2
10.764 ft^2	1 square meter	1 square foot	.093 m^2
.386 mi^2	1 square kilometer	1 square mile	2.59 km^2
2.47 ac	hectare	1 acre	.405 ha

Volume

Similarly, when measuring volume the relation between metric and standard units looks like this:

3034 fl oz	1 milliliter	1 fluid ounce	29.57 ml
.0264 gal	1 liter	1 gallon	3.785 L
35.314 ft^3	1 cubic meter	1 cubic foot	.028 m^3

Weight and Mass

When measuring weight and mass the relation between metric and standard units looks like this:

.035 oz	1 gram	1 ounce	28.35 g
2.202 lbs	1 kilogram	1 pound	.454 kg
1.103 T	1 metric ton	1 ton	.907 t

It is important to note that in science, the metric units of grams and kilograms are always used to denote the mass of an object rather than its weight.

In predominantly metric countries the standard unit of temperature is degrees Celsius while in countries with only limited use of the metric system, such as the United States, degrees Fahrenheit is used. This chart shows the difference between Fahrenheit and Celsius:

0° Celsius	32° Fahrenheit
10° Celsius	50° Fahrenheit
20° Celsius	68° Fahrenheit
30° Celsius	86° Fahrenheit
40° Celsius	104° Fahrenheit
50° Celsius	122° Fahrenheit
60° Celsius	140° Fahrenheit
70° Celsius	158° Fahrenheit
80° Celsius	176° Fahrenheit
90° Celsius	194° Fahrenheit
100° Celsius	212° Fahrenheit

As you can see, 0° C is freezing while 32° F is freezing. Similarity 100° C is boiling while the Fahrenheit system takes until 212° F. To convert from Celsius to Fahrenheit you need to multiply the temperature in Celsius by 1.8 and then add 32 to it. (x° F = (y° C*1.8) + 32) To convert from Fahrenheit to Celsius you do the opposite. First subtract 32 from the temperature then divide by 1.8. (x° C = (y° -32) / 1.8)

Exponents – a Quick Tutorial

Exponentiation is a mathematical operation, written as a^n, involving two numbers, the base, a, and the exponent (or power) n. When n is a positive integer, exponentiation corresponds to repeated multiplication; in other words, a product of n factors of a (the product itself can also be called power) just as multiplication by a positive integer corresponds to repeated addition.

The exponent is usually shown as a superscript to the right of the base. The exponentiation a^n can be read as: a raised to the n-th power, a raised to the power [of] n, or possibly raised to the exponent [of] n, or more briefly as a to the n. Some exponents have their own pronunciation: for example, a^2 is usually read as “a squared” and a^3 as “a cub ed.”

The power a^n can be defined also when n is a negative integer, for nonzero a.

Positive integer exponents

The expression $a^2 = a \cdot a$ is called the square of a because the area of a square with side-length a is a^2.

The expression $a^3 = a \cdot a \cdot a$ is called the cube, because the volume of a cube with side-length a, is a^3.

So 3^2 is pronounced "three squared," and 2^3 is "two cubed."

The exponent says how many copies of the base are multiplied together. For example, $3^5 = 3 \cdot 3 \cdot 3 \cdot 3 \cdot 3 = 243$. The base 3 appears 5 times in the repeated multiplication, because the exponent is 5. Here, 3 is the base, 5 is the exponent, or, more specifically, the fifth power of 3, 3 raised to the fifth power, or 3 to the power of 5.

The word "raised" is usually omitted, and very often "power" as well, so 3^5 is typically pronounced "three to the fifth" or "three to the five."

Exponents one and zero

Notice that a^1 is the "product" of only one a, which is defined to be a. Also note that $an^{-1} = a^n/a$. Assuming $n = 1$, we get $a^0 = 1$. Another way of saying this is that when n, m, and n^{-m} are positive (and if a is not equal to zero), one can see that

$a^n / a^m = a^{n-m}$

Extended to the special case when n and m are equal, the equality would read

$1 = a^n/a^n = a^{n-n} = a^0$

since both the numerator and the denominator are equal. Therefore we take this as the definition of a^0. This leads to the following rule:

Any number raised to the power 1 is the number itself.

Any nonzero number raised to the power 0 is 1; one interpretation of these powers is as empty products.

Negative integer exponents

By definition, raising a nonzero number to the −1 power produces its reciprocal:

$a^{-1} = 1/a$

One also defines

$a^{-n} = 1/ a^n$

for any nonzero a, and any positive integer n. Raising 0 to a negative power would imply division by 0, so it is left undefined.

The definition of a^{-n} for nonzero a is made so that the identity $a^m a^n = a^{m+n}$, initially true only for nonnegative integers m and n, holds for arbitrary integers m and n. In particular, requiring this identity for m = −n is requiring

$a^{-n} a^{n} = a^{-n+n} = a^0 = 1$

where a^0 is defined above, and this motivates the definition $a^{-n} = 1/an$ shown above.

Exponentiation to a negative integer power can alternatively be seen as repeated division of 1 by the base. For instance,

$3^{-4} = (((1/3)/3)/3)/3 = 1/81 = 1/3^4$

Identities and properties

The most important identity satisfied by integer exponentiation is $a^{m+n} = a^m \text{ X } a^n$

This identity has the consequence

$a^{m-n} = a^m / a^n$

for $a \neq 0$, and

$(a^m)^n = a^{M \text{ X } N}$

Another basic identity is

$(a + b)^n = a^n \text{ X } b^n$

While addition and multiplication are commutative (for example, 2+3 = 5 = 3+2 and 2·3 = 6 = 3·2), exponentiation is not commutative: $2^3 = 8$, but $3^2 = 9$.

Similarly, while addition and multiplication are associative (for example, (2+3)+4 = 9 = 2+(3+4) and (2·3)·4 = 24 = 2·(3·4), exponentiation is not associative either: 2^3 to the 4th power is 84 or 4096, but 2 to the 3^4 power is 281 or 2,417,851,639,229,258,349,412,3 52.

Powers of ten

In the base ten (decimal) number system, integer powers of 10 are written as the digit 1 followed or preceded by a number of zeroes determined by the sign and magnitude of the exponent. For example, $10^3 = 1000$ and $10^{-4} = 0.0001$.

Exponentiation with base 10 is used in scientific notation to describe large or small numbers. For instance, 299,792,458 meters/second (the speed of light in a vacuum, in meters per second) can be written as $2.99792458 \cdot 10^8$ m/s and then approximated as $2.998 \cdot 10^8$ m/s.

SI prefixes based on powers of 10 are also used to describe small or large quantities. For example, the prefix kilo means $10^3 = 1000$, so a kilometer is 1000 meters.

Fraction Tips, Tricks and Shortcuts

When you are writing an exam, time is precious, and anything you can do to answer questions faster, is a real advantage. Here are some ideas, shortcuts, tips and tricks that can speed up answering fraction problems.

Remember that a fraction is just a number which names a portion of something. For instance, instead of having a whole pie, a fraction says you have a part of a pie--such as a half of one or a fourth of one.

Two digits make up a fraction. The digit on top is known as the numerator. The digit on the bottom is known as the denominator. To remember which is which, just remember that "denominator" and "down" both start with a "d." And the "downstairs" number is the denominator. So for instance, in ½, the numerator is the 1 and the denominator (or "downstairs") number is the 2.

- It's easy to add two fractions if they have the same denominator. Just add the digits on top and leave the bottom one the same: 1/10 + 6/10 = 7/10.

- It's the same with subtracting fractions with the same denominator: 7/10 - 6/10 = 1/10.

- Adding and subtracting fractions with different denominators is a little more complicated. First, you have to get the problem so that they do have the same denominators. The easiest way to do this is to multiply the denominators: For 2/5 + 1/2 multiply 5 by 2. Now you have a denominator of 10. However, now you have to change the top numbers too. Since you multiplied the 5 in 2/5 by 2, you also multiply the 2 by 2, to get 4. So the first number is now 4/10. Since you multiplied the second number times 5, you also multiply its top number by 5, to get a final fraction of 5/10. Now you can add 5 and 4 together to get a final sum of 9/10.

- Sometimes you'll be asked to reduce a fraction to its simplest form. This means getting it to where the only common factor of the numerator and denominator is 1. Think of it this way: Numerators and denominators are brothers that must be treated the same. If you do something to one, you must do it to the other, or it's just not fair. For instance, if you divide your numerator by 2, then you should also divide the denominator by the same. Let's take an example: The fraction 2/10 . This is not reduced to its simplest terms because there is a number that will divide evenly into both: the number 2. We want to make it so that the only number that will divide evenly into both is 1. What can we divide into 2 to get 1? The number 2, of course! Now to be "fair," we have to do the same thing to the denominator: Divide 2 into 10 and you get 5. So our new, reduced fraction is 1/5.

- In some ways, multiplying fractions is the easiest of all: Just multiply the two top numbers and then multiply the two bottom numbers. For instance, with this problem:
  2/5 X 2/3 you multiply 2 by 2 and get a top number of 4; then multiply 5 by 3 and get a bottom number of 15. Your answer is 4/15.

- Dividing fractions is a bit more involved, but still not too hard. You once again multiply, but only AFTER you have turned the second fraction upside-down. To divide ⅞ by ½, turn the ½ into 2/1, then multiply the top numbers and multiply the bottom numbers: ⅞ X 2/1 gives us 14 on top and 8 on the bottom.

Converting Fractions to Decimals

There are a couple of ways to become good at converting fractions to decimals. One -- the one that will make you the fastest in basic math skills -- is to learn some basic fraction facts. It's a good idea, if you're good at memory, to memorize the following:

1/100 is "one hundredth," expressed as a decimal, it's .01.

1/50 is "two hundredths," expressed as a decimal, it's .02.

1/25 is "one twenty-fifths" or "four hundredths," expressed as a decimal, it's .04.

1/20 is "one twentieth" or ""five hundredths," expressed as a decimal, it's .05.

1/10 is "one tenth," expressed as a decimal, it's .1.

1/8 is "one eighth," or "one hundred twenty-five thousandths," expressed as a decimal, it's .125.

1/5 is "one fifth," or "two tenths," expressed as a decimal, it's .2.

1/4 is "one fourth" or "twenty-five hundredths," expressed as a decimal, it's .25.

1/3 is "one third" or "thirty-three hundredths," expressed as a decimal, it's .33.

1/2 is "one half" or "five tenths," expressed as a decimal, it's .5.

3/4 is "three fourths," or "seventy-five hundredths," expressed as a decimal, it's .75.

Of course, if you're no good at memorization, another good technique for converting a fraction to a decimal is to manipulate it so that the fraction's denominator is 10, 10,

1000, or some other power of 10. Here's an example: We'll start with ¾. What is the first number in the 4 "times table" that you can multiply and get a multiple of 10? Can you multiply 4 by something to get 10? No. Can you multiply it by something to get 100? Yes! 4 X 25 is 100. So let's take that 25 and multiply it by the numerator in our fraction ¾. The numerator is 3, and 3 X 25 is 75. We'll move the decimal in 75 all the way to the left, and we find that ¾ is .75.

We'll do another one: 1/5. Again, we want to find a power of 10 that 5 goes into evenly. Will 5 go into 10? Yes! It goes 2 times. So we'll take that 2 and multiply it by our numerator, 1, and we get 2. We move the decimal in 2 all the way to the left and find that 1/5 is equal to .2.

Converting Fractions to Percent

Working with either fractions or percents can be intimidating enough. But converting from one to the other? That's a genuine nightmare for those who are not math wizards. But really, it doesn't have to be that way. Here are two ways to make it easier and faster to convert a fraction to a percent.

- First, you might remember that a fraction is nothing more than a division problem: you're dividing the bottom number into the top number. So for instance, if we start with a fraction 1/10, we are making a division problem with the 10 on the outside the bracket and the 1 on the inside. As you remember from your lessons on dividing by decimals, since 10 won't go into 1, you add a decimal and make it 10 into 1.0. 10 into 10 goes 1 time, and since it's behind the decimal, it's .1. And how do we say .1? We say "one tenth," which is exactly what we started with: 1/10. So we have a number we can work with now: .1. When we're dealing with percents, though, we're dealing strictly with hundredths (not tenths). You remember from studying decimals that adding a zero to the right of the number on the right side of the decimal does not change the value. Therefore, we can change .1 into .10 and have the same number--except now it's expressed as hundredths. We have 10 hundredths. That's ten out of 100--which is just another way of saying ten percent (ten per hundred or ten out of 100). In other words .1 = .10 = 10 percent. Remember, if you're changing from a decimal to a percent, get rid of the decimal on the left and replace it with a percent mark on the right: 10%. Let's review those steps again: Divide 10 into 1. Since 10 doesn't go into 1, turn 1 into 1.0. Now divide 10 into 1.0. Since 10 goes into 10 1 time, put it there and add your decimal to make it .1. Since a percent is always "hundredths," let's change .1 into .10. Then remove the decimal on the left and replace with a percent sign on the right. The answer is 10%.

- If you're doing these conversions on a multiple-choice test, here's an idea that might be even easier and faster. Let's say you have a fraction of 1/8 and you're asked what the percent is. Since we know that "percent" means hundredths, ask yourself what number we can multiply 8 by to get 100. Since there is no number, ask what number gets us close to 100. That number is 12: 8 X 12 = 96. So it gets us a little less than 100. Now, whatever you do to the denominator, you have to do to the numerator. Let's multiply 1 X 12 and we get 12. However, since 96 is a little less than 100, we know that our answer will be a percent a little MORE than 12%. So if your possible answers on the multiple-choice test are these:

a) 8.5%   b) 19%   c)12.5%   d) 25%

then we know the answer is c) 12.5%, because it's a little MORE than the 12 we got in our math problem above.

Another way to look at this, using multiple choice strategy is you know the answer will be "about" 12. Looking at the other choices, they are all too large or too small and can be eliminated right away.

This was an easy example to demonstrate, so don't be fooled! You probably won't get such an easy question on your exam, but the principle holds just the same. By estimating your answer quickly, you can eliminate choices immediately and save precious exam time.

Decimal Tips, Tricks and Shortcuts

Converting Decimals to Fractions

One of the most important tricks for correctly converting a decimal to a fraction doesn't involve math at all. It's simply to learn to say the decimal correctly. If you say "point one" or "point 25" for .1 and .25, you'll have more trouble getting the conversion correct. But if you know that it's called "one tenth" and "twenty-five hundredths," you're on the way to a correct conversion. That's because, if you know your fractions, you know that "one tenth" looks like this: 1/10. And "twenty-five hundredths" looks like this: 25/100.

Even if you have digits before the decimal, such as 3.4, learning how to say the word will help you with the conversion into a fraction. It's not "three point four," it's "three and four tenths." Knowing this, you know that the fraction which looks like "three and four tenths" is 3 4/10.

Of course, your conversion is not complete until you reduce the fraction to its lowest terms: It's not 25/100, but 1/4.

Converting Decimals to Percent

Changing a decimal to a percent is easy if you remember one math formula: multiply by 100. For instance, if you start with .45, you change it to a percent by simply multiplying it by 100. You then wind up with 45. Add the % sign to the end and you get 45%.

That seems easy enough, right? Here think of it this way: You just take out the decimal and stick in a percent sign on the opposite sign. In other words, the decimal on the left is replaced by the % on the right.

It doesn't work quite that easily if the decimal is in the middle of the number. Let's use 3.7 for example. Here, take out the decimal in the middle and replace it with a 0 % at the end. So 3.7 converted to decimal is 370%.

Percent Tips, Tricks and Shortcuts

Percent problems are not nearly as scary as they appear, if you remember this neat trick:

Draw a cross as in:

Portion	Percent
Whole	100

In the upper left, write PORTION. In the bottom left, write WHOLE. In the top right, write PERCENT and in the bottom right, write 100. Whatever your problem is, you will leave blank the unknown, and fill in the other four parts. For example, let's suppose your problem is: Find 10% of 50. Since we know the 10% part, we put 10 in the percent corner. Since the whole number in our problem is 50, we put that in the corner marked whole. You always put 100 underneath the percent, so we leave it as is, which leaves only the top left corner blank. This is where we'll put our answer. Now simply multiply the two corner numbers that are NOT 100. Here, it's 10 X 50. That gives us 500. Now multiply this by the remaining corner, or 100, to get a final answer of 5. 5 is the number that goes in the upper-left corner, and is your final solution.
Another hint to remember: Percents are the same thing as hundredths in decimals. So .45 is the same as 45 hundredths or 45 percent.

Converting Percents to Decimals

Percents are simply a specific type of decimals, so it should be no surprise that converting between the two is actually fairly simple. Here are a few tricks and shortcuts to keep in mind:

- Remember that percent literally means "per 100" or "for every 100." So when you speak of 30% you're saying 30 for every 100 or the fraction 30/100. In basic math, you learned that fractions that have 10 or 100 as the denominator can easily be turned into a decimal. 30/100 is thirty hundredths, or expressed as a decimal, .30.

- Another way to look at it: To convert a percent to a decimal, simply divide the number by 100. So for instance, if the percent is 47%, divide 47 by 100. The result will be .47. Get rid of the % mark and you're done.
- Remember that the easiest way of dividing by 100 is by moving your decimal two spots to the left.

Converting Percents to Fractions

Converting percents to fractions is easy. After all, a percent is nothing except a type of fraction; it tells you what part of 100 that you're talking about. Here are some simple ideas for making the conversion from a percent to a fraction:

- If the percent is a whole number -- say 34% -- then simply write a fraction with 100 as the denominator (the bottom number). Then put the percentage itself on top. So 34% becomes 34/100.
- Now reduce as you would reduce any percent. Here, by dividing 2 into 34 and 2 into 100, you get 17/50.
- If your percent is not a whole number -- say 3.4% --then convert it to a decimal expressed as hundredths. 3.4 is the same as 3.40 (or 3 and forty hundredths). Now ask yourself how you would express "three and forty hundredths" as a fraction. It would, of course, be 3 40/100. Reduce this and it becomes 3 2/5.

How to Answer Basic Math Multiple Choice

Math is the one section where you need to make sure that you understand the processes before you ever tackle it. That's because the time allowed on the math portion is typically so short that there's not much room for error. You have to be fast and accurate. It's imperative that before the test day arrives, you've learned all the main formulas that will be used, and then to create your own problems (and solve them).

On the actual test day, use the "Plug-Check-Check" strategy. Here's how it goes.

Read the problem, but not the answers. You'll want to work the problem first and come up with your own answers. If you did the work right, you should find your answer among the options given.

If you need help with the problem, plug actual numbers into the variables given. You'll find it easier to work with numbers than it is to work with letters. For instance, if the question asks, "If Y-4 is 2 more than Z, then Y+5 is how much more than Z?" try selecting a value for Y. Let's take 6. Your question now becomes, "If 6-4 is 2 more than Z, then 6 plus 5 is how much more than Z?" Now your answer should be easier to work with.

Check the answer options to see if your answer matches one of those. If so, select it.

If no answer matches the one you got, re-check your math, but this time, use a different method. In math, it's common for there to be more than one way to solve a problem. As a simple example, if you multiplied 12 X 13 and did not get an answer that matches one of the answer options, you might try adding 13 together 12 different times and see if you get a good answer.

Math Multiple Choice Strategy

The two strategies for working with basic math multiple choice are Estimation and Elimination.

Math Strategy 1 - Estimation.

Just like it sounds, try to estimate an approximate answer first. Then look at the choices.

Math Strategy 2 - Elimination.

For every question, no matter what type, eliminating obviously incorrect answers narrows the possible choices. Elimination is probably the most powerful strategy for answering multiple choice.

Here are a few basic math examples of how this works.

Solve 2/3 + 5/12

a. 9/17

b. 3/11

c. 7/12

d. 1 1/12

First estimate the answer. 2/3 is more than half and 5/12 is about half, so the answer is going to be very close to 1.

Next, Eliminate. Choice A is about 1/2 and can be eliminated, Choice B is very small, less than 1/2 and can be eliminated. Choice C is close to 1/2 and can be eliminated. Leaving only Choice D, which is just over 1.

Work through the solution, a common denominator is needed, a number which both 3 and 12 will divide into.
2/3 = 8/12. So, 8+5/12 = 13/12 = 1 1/12

Choice D is correct.

Solve 4/5 - 2/3

a. 2/2
b. 2/13
c. 1
d. 2/15

You can eliminate Choice A, because it is 1 and since both of the numbers are close to one, the difference is going to be very small. You can eliminate Choice C for the same reason.

Next, look at the denominators. Since 5 and 3 don't go into 13, you can eliminate Choice B as well.

That leaves Choice D.

Checking the answer, the common denominator will be 15. So 12-10/15 = 2/15. Choice D is correct.

Fractions shortcut - Cancelling out.

In any operation with fractions, if the numerator of one fraction has a common multiple with the denominator of the other, you can cancel out. This saves time and simplifies the problem quickly, making it easier to manage.

Solve 2/15 ÷ 4/5

a. 6/65
b. 6/75
c. 5/12
d. 1/6

To divide fractions, we multiply the first fraction with the inverse of the second fraction. Therefore we have
2/15 x 5/4. The numerator of the first fraction, 2, shares a multiple with the denominator of the second fraction, 4, which is 2. These cancel out, which gives, 1/3 x 1/2 = 1/6

Cancelling Out solved the questions very quickly, but we can still use multiple choice strategies to answer.

Choice B can be eliminated because 75 is too large a denominator. Choice C can be eliminated because 5 and 15 don't go into 12.

Choice D is correct.

Decimal Multiple Choice strategy and Shortcuts.

Multiplying decimals gives a very quick way to estimate and eliminate choices. Any-time that you multiply decimals, it is going to give an answer with the same number of decimal places as the combined operands.

So for example,

2.38 X 1.2 will produce a number with three places of decimal, which is 2.856.

Here are a few examples with step-by-step explanation:

Solve 2.06 x 1.2

a. 24.82

b. 2.482

c. 24.72

d. 2.472

This is a simple question, but even before you start calculating, you can eliminate several choices. When multiplying decimals, there will always be as many numbers behind the decimal place in the answer as the sum of the ones in the initial problem, so Choice A and C can be eliminated.

The correct answer is D: 2.06 x 1.2 = 2.472

Solve 20.0 ÷ 2.5

a. 12.05

b. 9.25

c. 8.3

d. 8

First estimate the answer to be around 10, and eliminate Choice A. And since it'd also be an even number, you can eliminate Choice B and C., leaving only choice D.

The correct Answer is D: 20.0 ÷ 2.5 = 8

How to Solve Word Problems

Most students find math word problems difficult. Tackling word problems is much easier if you have a systematic approach which we outline below.

Here is the biggest tip for studying word problems.

Practice regularly and systematically. Sounds simple and easy right? Yes it is, and yes it really does work.

Word problems are a way of thinking and require you to translate a real word problem into mathematical terms.

Some math instructors go so far as to say that learning how to think mathematically is the main reason for teaching word problems.

So what do we mean by Practice regularly and systematically? Studying word problems and math in general requires a logical and mathematical frame of mind. The only way you can get this is by practicing regularly, which means everyday.

It is critical that you practice word problems everyday for the 5 days before the exam as a bare minimum.

If you practice and miss a day, you have lost the mathematical frame of mind and the benefit of your previous practice is pretty much gone. Anyone who has done any amount of math will agree – you have to practice everyday.

Everything is important. The other critical point about word problems is that all of the information given in the problem has some purpose. There is no unnecessary information! Word problems are typically around 50 words in 1 to 3 sentences. If the sometimes complicated relationships are to be explained in that short an explanation, every word has to count. Make sure that you use every piece of information.

Here are 9 simple steps to help you resolve word problems.

Step 1 – Read through the problem at least three times. The first reading should be a quick scan, and the next two readings should be done slowly with a view to finding answers to these important questions:

What does the problem ask? (Usually located towards the end of the problem)

What does the problem imply? (This is usually a point you were asked to remember).

Mark all information, and underline all important words or phrases.

Step 2 – Try to make a pictorial representation of the problem such as a circle and an arrow to show travel. This makes the problem a bit more real and sensible to you.

A favorite word problem is something like, 1 train leaves Station A travelling at 100 km/hr and another train leaves Station B travelling at 60 km/hr. ...

Draw a line, the two stations, and the two trains at either end. This will help solidify the situation in your mind.

Step 3 – Use the information you have to make a table with a blank portion to show information you do not know.

Step 4 – Assign a single letter to represent each unknown data in your table. You can write down the unknown that each letter represents so that you do not make the error of assigning answers to the wrong unknown, because a word problem may have multiple unknowns and you will need to create equations for each unknown.

Step 5 – Translate the English terms in the word problem into a mathematical algebraic equation. Remember that the main problem with word problems is that they are not expressed in regular math equations. You ability to correctly identify the variables and translate the word problem into an equation determines your ability to solve the problem.

Step 6 – Check the equation to see if it looks like regular equations that you are used to seeing and whether it looks sensible. Does the equation appear to represent the information in the question? Take note that you may need to rewrite some formulas needed to solve the word problem equation. For example, word distance problems may need rewriting the distance formula, which is Distance = Time x Rate. If the word problem requires that you solve for time you will need to use Distance/Rate and Distance/Time to solve for Rate. If you understand the distance word problem you should be able to identify the variable you need to solve for.

Step 7 – Use algebra rules to solve the derived equation. Take note that the laws of equation demands that what is done on this side of the equation has to also be done on the other side. You have to solve the equation so that the unknown ends up alone on one side. Where there are multiple unknowns you will need to use elimination or substitution methods to resolve all the equations.

Step 8 – Check your final answers to see if they make sense with the information given in the problem. For example if the word problem involves a discount, the final price should be less or if a product was taxed then the final answer has to cost more.

Step 9 – Cross check your answers by placing the answer or answers in the first equation to replace the unknown or unknowns. If your answer is correct then both side of the equation must equate or equal. If your answer is not correct then you may have derived a wrong equation or solved the equation wrongly. Repeat the necessary steps to correct.

Types of Word Problems

Word problems can be classified into 12 types. Below are examples of each type with a complete solution. Some types of word problems can be solved quickly using multiple choice strategies and some can not. Always look for ways to estimate the answer and then eliminate choices.

1. Age

A girl is 10 years older than her brother. By next year, she will be twice the age of her brother. What are their ages now?

a. 25, 15
b. 19, 9
c. 21, 11
d. 29, 19

Solution: B

We will assume that the girl's age is "a" and her brother's is "b." This means that based on the information in the first sentence,
$a = 10 + b$

Next year, she will be twice her brother's age, which gives
$a + 1 = 2(b+1)$

We need to solve for one unknown factor and then use the answer to solve for the other. To do this we substitute the value of "a" from the first equation into the second equation. This gives

$10+b + 1 = 2b + 2$
$11 + b = 2b + 2$
$11 - 2 = 2b - b$
$b= 9$

$9 = b$ this means that her brother is 9 years old. Solving for the girl's age in the first equation gives $a = 10 + 9$. $a = 19$ the girl is aged 19. So, the girl is aged 19 and the boy is 9

2. Distance or speed

Two boats travel down a river towards the same destination, starting at the same time. One boat is traveling at 52 km/hr, and the other boat at 43 km/hr. How far apart will they be after 40 minutes?

a. 46.67 km
b. 19.23 km
c. 6.4 km
d. 14.39 km

Solution: C

After 40 minutes, the first boat will have traveled = 52 km/hr x 40 minutes/60 minutes = 34.7 km

After 40 minutes, the second boat will have traveled = 43 km/hr x 40/60 minutes = 28.66 km
Difference between the two boats will be 34.7 km – 28.66 km = 6.04 km.

Multiple Choice Strategy

First estimate the answer. The first boat is travelling 9 km. faster than the second, for 40 minutes, which is 2/3 of an hour. 2/3 of 9 = 6, as a rough guess of the distance apart.

Choices A, B and D can be eliminated right away.

3. Ratio

The instructions in a cookbook states that 700 grams of flour must be mixed in 100 ml of water, and 0.90 grams of salt added. A cook however has just 325 grams of flour. What is the quantity of water and salt that he should use?

a. 0.41 grams and 46.4 ml
b. 0.45 grams and 49.3 ml
c. 0.39 grams and 39.8 ml
d. 0.25 grams and 40.1 ml

Solution: A

The Cookbook states 700 grams of flour, but the cook only has 325. The first step is to determine the percentage of flour he has 325/700 x 100 = 46.4%
That means that 46.4% of all other items must also be used.
46.4% of 100 = 46.4 ml of water
46.4% of 0.90 = 0.41 grams of salt.

Multiple Choice Strategy

The recipe calls for 700 grams of flour but the cook only has 325, which is just less than half, the amount of water and salt are going to be about half.

Choices C and D can be eliminated right away. Choice B is very close so be careful. Looking closely at Choice B, it is exactly half, and since 325 is slightly less than half of 700, it can't be correct.

Choice A is correct.

4. Percent

An agent received $6,685 as his commission for selling a property. If his commission was 13% of the selling price, how much was the property?

a. $68,825
b. $121,850
c. $49,025
d. $51,423

Solution: D

Let's assume that the property price is x
That means from the information given, 13% of x = 6,685
Solve for x,
x = 6685 x 100/13 = $51,423

Multiple Choice Strategy

The commission,13%, is just over 10%, which is easier to work with. Round up $6685 to $6700, and multiple by 10 for an approximate answer. 10 X 6700 = $67,000. You can do this in your head. Choice B is much too big and can be eliminated. Choice C is too small and can be eliminated. Choices A and D are left and good possibilities.

Do the calculations to make the final choice.

5. Sales & Profit

A store owner buys merchandise for $21,045. He transports them for $3,905 and pays his staff $1,450 to stock the merchandise on his shelves. If he does not incur further costs, how much does he need to sell the items to make $5,000 profit?

a. $32,500
b. $29,350
c. $32,400
d. $31,400

Solution: D

Total cost of the items is $21,045 + $3,905 + $1,450 = $26,400
Total cost is now $26,400 + $5000 profit = $31,400

Multiple Choice Strategy

Round off and add the numbers up in your head quickly.
21,000 + 4,000 + 1500 = 26500. Add in 5000 profit for a total of 31500.

Choice B is too small and can be eliminated. Choice C and Choice A are too large and can be eliminated.

6. Tax/Income

A woman earns $42,000 per month and pays 5% tax on her monthly income. If the Government increases her monthly taxes by $1,500, what is her income after tax?

a. $38,400
b. $36,050
c. $40,500
d. $39, 500

Solution: A

Initial tax on income was 5/100 x 42,000 = $2,100
$1,500 was added to the tax to give $2,100 + 1,500 = $3,600
Income after tax left is $42,000 - $3,600 = $38,400

7. Interest

A man invests $3000 in a 2-year term deposit that pays 3% interest per year. How much will he have at the end of the 2-year term?

a. $5,200
b. $3,020
c. $3,182.7
d. $3,000

Solution: C

This is a compound interest problem. The funds are invested for 2 years and interest is paid yearly, so in the second year, he will earn interest on the interest paid in the first year.

3% interest in the first year = 3/100 x 3,000 = $90
At end of first year, total amount = 3,000 + 90 = $3,090
Second year = 3/100 x 3,090 = 92.7.
At end of second year, total amount = $3090 + $92.7 = $3,182.7

8. Averaging

The average weight of 10 books is 54 grams. 2 more books were added and the average weight became 55.4. If one of the 2 new books added weighed 62.8 g, what is the weight of the other?

a. 44.7 g
b. 67.4 g
c. 62 g
d. 52 g

Solution: C

Total weight of 10 books with average 54 grams will be=10×54=540 g
Total weight of 12 books with average 55.4 will be=55.4×12=664.8 g
So total weight of the remaining 2 will be= 664.8 – 540 = 124.8 g
If one weighs 62.8, the weight of the other will be= 124.8 g – 62.8 g = 62 g

Multiple Choice Strategy

Averaging problems can be estimated by looking at which direction the average goes. If additional items are added and the average goes up, the new items much be greater than the average. If the average goes down after new items are added, the new items must be less than the average.

Here, the average is 54 grams and 2 books are added which increases the average to 55.4, so the new books must weight more than 54 grams.

Choices A and D can be eliminated right away.

9. Probability

A bag contains 15 marbles of various colors. If 3 marbles are white, 5 are red and the rest are black, what is the probability of randomly picking out a black marble from the bag?

a. 7/15
b. 3/15
c. 1/5
d. 4/15

Solution: A

Total marbles = 15
Number of black marbles = 15 – (3 + 5) = 7
Probability of picking out a black marble = 7/15

10. Two Variables

A company paid a total of $2850 to book for 6 single rooms and 4 double rooms in a hotel for one night. Another company paid $3185 to book for 13 single rooms for one night in the same hotel. What is the cost for single and double rooms in that hotel?

a. single= $250 and double = $345
b. single= $254 and double = $350
c. single = $245 and double = $305
d. single = $245 and double = $345

Solution: D

We can determine the price of single rooms from the information given of the second company. 13 single rooms = 3185.
One single room = 3185 / 13 = 245
The first company paid for 6 single rooms at $245. 245 x 6 = $1470
Total amount paid for 4 double rooms by first company = $2850 - $1470 = $1380
Cost per double room = 1380 / 4 = $345

11. Geometry

The length of a rectangle is 5 in. more than its width. The perimeter of the rectangle is 26 in. What is the width and length of the rectangle?

a. width = 6 inches, Length = 9 inches
b. width = 4 inches, Length = 9 inches
c. width =4 inches, Length = 5 inches
d. width = 6 inches, Length = 11 inches

Solution: B

Formula for perimeter of a rectangle is 2(L + W)
p=26, so 2(L+W) = p
The length is 5 inches more than the width, so
2(w+5) + 2w = 26
2w + 10 + 2w = 26
2w + 2w = 26 - 10
4w = 16

W = 16/4 = 4 inches

L is 5 inches more than w, so L = 5 + 4 = 9 inches.

12. Totals and fractions

A basket contains 125 oranges, mangos and apples. If 3/5 of the fruits in the basket are mangos and only 2/5 of the mangos are ripe, how many ripe mangos are there in the basket?

a. 30
b. 68
c. 55
d. 47

Solution: A
Number of mangos in the basket is 3/5 x 125 = 75
Number of ripe mangos = 2/5 x 75 = 30
5
Number of ripe mangos = 2/5 x 75 = 30

English

THIS SECTION CONTAINS A SELF-ASSESSMENT AND ENGLISH TUTORIALS. The Tutorials are designed to familiarize general principles and the Self-Assessment contains general questions similar to the English questions likely to be on the DET exam, but are not intended to be identical to the exam questions. Many Universities recommend that students take an introductory English course before taking the DET Exam. The tutorials are *not* designed to be a complete English course, and it is assumed that students have some familiarity with English. If you do not understand parts of the tutorial, or find the tutorial difficult, it is recommended that you seek out additional instruction.

The purpose of the self-assessment is:

- Identify your strengths and weaknesses.
- Develop your personalized study plan (above)
- Get accustomed to the DET format
- Extra practice – the self-assessment is a 3rd test!

Since this is a self-assessment, and depending on how confident you are with English Grammar, timing yourself is optional. There are a total of 50 questions which must be answered in 50 minutes. The self-assessment has 20 questions, so allow 20 minutes to complete this assessment.

The questions below are not the same as you will find on the DET - that would be too easy! And nobody knows what the questions will be and they change all the time. Below are general English questions that cover the same areas as the DET. So the format and exact wording of the questions may differ slightly, and change from year to year, if you can answer the questions below, you will have no problem with the English section of the DET.

NOTE: The English section is an optional module and not all schools include in their DET. We strongly suggest that you check with your school for the DET exam details. It is always a good idea to give the materials you receive when you register to take the DET a careful review.

75% - 100%	Excellent – you have mastered the content
50 – 75%	Good. You have a working knowledge. Even though you can just pass this section, you may want to review the Tutorials and do some extra practice to see if you can improve your mark.
25% - 50%	Below Average. You do not understand the content. Review the tutorials, and retake this quiz again in a few days, before proceeding to the rest of the practice test questions.
Less than 25%	Poor. You have a very limited understanding. Please review the Tutorials, and retake this quiz again in a few days, before proceeding to the rest of the practice test questions.

English Self-Assessment Answer Sheet

1. (A) (B) (C) (D)
2. (A) (B) (C) (D)
3. (A) (B) (C) (D)
4. (A) (B) (C) (D)
5. (A) (B) (C) (D)
6. (A) (B) (C) (D)
7. (A) (B) (C) (D)
8. (A) (B) (C) (D)
9. (A) (B) (C) (D)
10. (A) (B) (C) (D)

1. Choose the sentence with the correct grammar.

a. He would have postponed the camping trip, if he would have known about the forecast.

b. If he would have known about the forecast, he would have postponed the camping trip.

c. If he have known about the forecast, he would have postponed the camping trip.

d. If he had known about the forecast, he would have postponed the camping trip.

2. Choose the sentence with the correct grammar.

a. If Joe had told me the truth, I wouldn't have been so angry.

b. If Joe would have told me the truth, I wouldn't have been so angry.

c. I wouldn't have been so angry if Joe would have told the truth.

d. If Joe would have telled me the truth, I wouldn't have been so angry.

3. Choose the sentence with the correct grammar.

a. He doesn't have any money to buy clothes, and neither do I.

b. He doesn't have any money to buy clothes, and neither does I.

c. He don't have any money to buy clothes, and neither do I.

d. He don't have any money to buy clothes, and neither does I.

4. Choose the sentence with the correct grammar.

a. Because it really don't matter, I don't care if I go there.

b. Because it really doesn't matter, I doesn't care if I go there.

c. Because it really doesn't matter, I don't care if I go there.

d. Because it really don't matter, I don't care if I go there.

5. Choose the sentence with the correct grammar.

a. The dog took the stuffed toy to his master's empty chair.

b. The dog brang the stuffed toy to his master's empty chair.

c. The dog brought the stuffed toy to his master's empty chair.

d. The dog taken the stuffed toy to his master's empty chair.

6. Choose the sentence with the correct grammar.

a. Until you take the overdue books to the library, you can't take any new ones home.

b. Until you take the overdue books to the library, you can't bring any new ones home.

c. Until you bring the overdue books to the library, you can't take any new ones home.

d. Until you take the overdue books to the library, you can't take any new ones home.

7. Choose the sentence with the correct grammar.

a. Newer cars use fewer gasoline and produce fewer emissions.

b. Newer cars use less gasoline and produce less emissions.

c. Newer cars use less gasoline and produce fewer emissions.

d. Newer cars fewer less gasoline and produce less emissions.

8. Choose the sentence with the correct grammar.

a. His doctor suggested that he eat less snacks and do fewer lounging on the couch.

b. His doctor suggested that he eat fewer snacks and do less lounging on the couch.

c. His doctor suggested that he eat less snacks and do less lounging on the couch.

d. His doctor suggested that he eat fewer snacks and do fewer lounging on the couch.

9. Choose the sentence with the correct grammar.

a. However, I believe that he didn't really try that hard.

b. However I believe that he didn't really try that hard.

c. However; I believe that he didn't really try that hard.

d. However: I believe that he didn't really try that hard.

10. Choose the sentence with the correct grammar.

a. There was however, very little difference between the two.

b. There was, however very little difference between the two.

c. There was; however, very little difference between the two.

d. There was, however, very little difference between the two.

Answer Key

1. D

The third conditional is used for talking about an unreal situation (a situation that did not happen) in the past. For example, “If I had studied harder, [if clause] I would have passed the exam [main clause]. This has the same meaning as, “I failed the exam because I didn’t study hard enough.”

2. A

The third conditional is used for talking about an unreal situation (a situation that did not happen) in the past. For example, “If I had studied harder, [if clause] I would have passed the exam [main clause]. This has the same meaning as, “I failed the exam because I didn’t study hard enough.”

3. A

Shows agreement with a negative statement by using “neither.”

4. C

Doesn’t, does not, or does is used with the third person singular--the pronouns he, she, and it. Don’t, do not, or do is used with first, second, and third person plural.

5. A

Whether to use “bring” or “take” depends on location. Something coming toward the subject’s location is brought. Something going away from the subject’s location is taken.

6. C

Whether to use “bring” or “take” depends on location. Something coming toward the subject’s location is brought. Something going away from the subject’s location is taken.

7. C

“Fewer” is used with countable nouns and “less” is used with uncountable nouns.

8. B

“Fewer” is used with countable nouns and “less” is used with uncountable nouns.

9. A

“However” is bracketed with a comma after it at the beginning of a sentence.

10. D

“However” is bracketed with a comma before and after it within a sentence.

English Tutorials

Included in this section:

Independent Clauses and Coordinating Conjunctions

Capitalization

Types of Sentences

Verb Tenses

Verb Types - Transitive, Intransitive and Linking

Punctuation

- Colons
- Semicolons
- Hyphens
- Dashes
- Parentheses
- Apostrophes
- Commas
- Quotation Marks

English Grammar and Punctuation Tutorials

Capitalization

Although many of the rules for capitalization are pretty straight forward, there are several tricky points that are important to review.

Starting a Sentence

Everyone knows that you need to capitalize the first letter of the first word in a sentence, but is it really all that easy to figure out where one sentence starts and another stops? Take these three examples:

That was the moment it really sunk in: There would be no hockey this year.

It was April and that could mean only one thing: baseball.

We played for hours before heading home; everyone felt tired and happy.

In the first example, the first letter after the colon is capitalized while in the second example it is not. That is because everything after the first example's colon is a complete sentence, while after example two's colon there is only one word. In example three you have what could be a complete sentence ("everyone felt tired and happy"), but which is not because it follows a semicolon, making it just another clause instead.

Within a sentence you can have an additional complete sentence if the sentence follows a colon. But if what could be a complete sentence follows a semicolon, it is a clause and does not get capitalized.

Remember that the same rules apply for quotation marks that apply for colons: A complete sentence inside quotation marks is capitalized, but a single word or phrase is not.

Proper Nouns

The first letter of all proper nouns needs to be capitalized. There are many categories of proper noun. The most common proper nouns are the specific names of people (such as Bill), places (such as Germany) or things (such as Honda Civic). However, there are several less obvious categories of words that should be capitalized as proper nouns.

Historical events such as World War II or the California Gold Rush need to be capitalized.

The names of celestial bodies such as Orion's Belt need to be capitalized.

The names of ethnicities such as African-American or Hispanic need to be capitalized.

Relationship words that replace a person's name such as Mom, Doctor and Mister need to be capitalized. However, this only happens when you use the word to replace the person's name. In the sentence, "My mom went to the store," you do not capitalize it, while in the sentence, "Hey Mom, did you get toothpaste at the store?" you do capitalize it.

Geographical locations are capitalized. This can get a little tricky because capitalized geographical locations and non-capitalized directions are easy to confuse. Saying, "We drove south for hours," is a direction, so the word "south" should not be capitalized. But when saying, "While in the United States, we drove to the South to look at Civil War battle fields," you do capitalize the word "South." The difference is that in the first sentence "south" is just the direction you drove. In the second sentence "the South" is a specific region of the United States that formed itself into the Confederacy during the US Civil War.

Proper Adjectives

Proper adjectives are the adjective forms of proper nouns. People from Germany are German; people from Canada are Canadian. German and Canadian are proper adjectives because they are forms of proper nouns that are used to describe other nouns.

Titles of Works

Titles of works are generally capitalized following a specific pattern. Capitalize all of the important words in a sentence. Do not capitalize unimportant words such as prepositions and articles.

For example: Alien Spaceship Spotted over Many of the World's Capitals

Notice that the prepositions "over" and "of," and the article "the" are the only non-capitalized words in the sentence.

Colons and Semicolons

Within a sentence there are several different types of punctuation marks that can denote a pause. Each of these punctuation marks has different rules when it comes to its structure and usage, so we will look at each one in turn.

Colons

The colon is used primarily to introduce information. It can start lists such as in the sentence, "There were several things Susan had to get at the store: bread, cereal, lettuce and tomatoes." Or a colon points out specific information, such as in the sentence, "It was only then that the group fully realized what had happened: The Martian invasion had begun."

Note that if the information after the colon is a complete sentence, you capitalize and punctuate it exactly like you would a sentence. If, however, it does not constitute a complete sentence, you don't have to capitalize anything. ("Peering out the window Meredith saw them: zombies.")

Semicolons

Semicolons can be thought of as super commas. They denote a stronger stop than a comma does, but they are still weaker than a period, not quite capable of ending a sentence. Semicolons are primarily used to separate independent clauses that are not being separated by a coordinating conjunction. ("Chris went to the store; he bought chips and salsa.") Semicolons can only do this, however, when the ideas in each clause are related. For instance, the sentence, "It's raining outside; my sister went to the movies," is not a proper usage of the semicolon since those clauses have nothing to do with each other.

Semicolons can also be used in lists if one or more element in the list is itself made up of a smaller list. If you want to write a list of things you plan to bring to a picnic, and those things only include a Frisbee, a chair and some pasta salad, you would not need to use a semicolon. However, if you also wanted to bring plastic knives, forks and spoons, you would need to write your sentence like this: "For our picnic I am bringing a Frisbee; a chair; plastic knives, forks and spoons; and some pasta salad."

Using semicolons like this preserves the smaller list that you have in your larger list.

Commas

Commas are probably the most commonly used punctuation mark in English. Commas can break the flow of writing to give it a more natural sounding style, and they are the main punctuation mark used to separate ideas. Commas also separate lists, introductory adverbs, introductory prepositional phrases, dates and addresses.

The most rigid way that commas are used is when separating clauses. There are two primary types of clauses in a sentence, independent and subordinate (sometimes called dependent). Independent clauses are clauses that express a complete thought, such as, "Tim went to the store." Subordinate clauses, on the other hand, only express partial thoughts that expand on an independent clause, such as, "after the game ended," which you can see is clearly not a complete sentence. (You will learn more about clauses in different lessons.)

The rule for commas with clauses is that a comma must separate the clauses when a subordinate clause comes first in a sentence: "After the game ended, Tim went to the store." But there should not be a comma when a subordinate clause follows an independent clause: "Tim went to the store after the game ended." If you leave the comma out of the first example, you have a run-on sentence. If you add one into the second example, you have a comma-splice error. Also, when you have two independent clauses joined with a coordinating conjunction, you need to separate them with a comma. "Tim went to the store, and Beth went home."

There are some artistic exceptions to these rules, such as adding a pause for literary effect, but for the most part they are set in stone.

Commas are also used to separate items in a list. This area of English is unfortunately less clear than it should be, with two separate rules depending on what standard you are following. To understand the two different rules, let's pretend you are having a party at your house, and you are making a list of refreshments your friends will want. You may decide to serve three things: 1) pizza 2) chips 3) drinks. There are two different rules governing how you should punctuate this. According to many grammar books, you would write this as, "At the store I will buy pizza, chips, and drinks." This variation puts a comma after each item in the list. It is the version that the style books used in most college English and history courses will prefer, so it is probably the one you should follow. However, the Associated Press style guide, which is used in college journalism classes and at newspapers and magazines, says the sentence should be written like this: "At the store I will buy pizza, chips and drinks." Here you only use a comma between the first two words, letting the word "and" act as the separator between the last two.

Another important place to use commas is when you have a modifier that describes an element of a sentence, but that does not directly follow the thing it describes. Look at the sentence: "Tim went over to visit Beth, watching the full moon along the way." In this sentence there is no confusion about who is "watching the full moon"; it is Tim, probably as he walks to Beth's house. If you remove the comma, however, you get this: "Tim went over to visit Beth watching the full moon along the way." Now it sounds as though Beth is watching the full moon, and we are forced to wonder what "way" the moon is traveling along.

Commas are also used when adding introductory prepositional phrases and introductory adverbs to sentences. A comma is always needed following an introductory adverb. ("Quickly, Jody ran to the car.") Commas are even necessary when you have an adverb introducing a clause within a sentence, even if the clause not the first clause of the sentence. ("Amanda wanted to go to the movie; however, she knew her homework was more important.")

With introductory prepositional phrases you only add a comma if the phrase (or if a group of introductory phrases) is five or more words long. Thus, the sentence you just read did not have a comma following its introductory prepositional phrase ("With introductory prepositional phrases") because it was only four words. Compare that to this sentence with a five word introductory phrase: "After the ridiculously long class, the friends needed to relax."

The last main way that commas are used in sentences is to separate out information that does not need to be there. For instance, "My cousin Hector, who wore a blue hat at the party, thought you were funny." The fact that Hector wore a blue hat is interesting, but it is not vital to the sentence; it could be removed and not changed the sentence's meaning. Therefore, it gets commas around it. Along these lines you should remember that any clause introduced by the word that is considered to provide essential information to the sentence and should not get commas around it. Conversely, any clause starting with the word which is considered nonessential and should not get commas around it.

How to Answer English Grammar Multiple Choice - Verb Tense

This tutorial is designed to help you answer English Grammar multiple choice questions as well as a very quick refresher on verb tenses. It is assumed that you have some familiarity with the verb tenses covered here. If you find these questions difficulty or do not understand the tense construction, we recommend you seek out additional instruction.

Tenses Covered

1. Past Progressive
2. Present Perfect
3. Present Perfect Progressive
4. Present Progressive
5. Simple Future
6. Simple Future – "Going to" Form
7. Past Perfect Progressive
8. Future Perfect Progressive
9. Future Perfect
10. Future Progressive
11. Past Perfect

1. The Past Progressive Tense

How to Recognize This Tense

He *was running* very fast when he fell.

They *were drinking* coffee when he arrived.

About the Past Progressive Tense

This tense is used to speak of an action that was in progress in the past when another event occurred.

The action was unfolding at a point in the past.

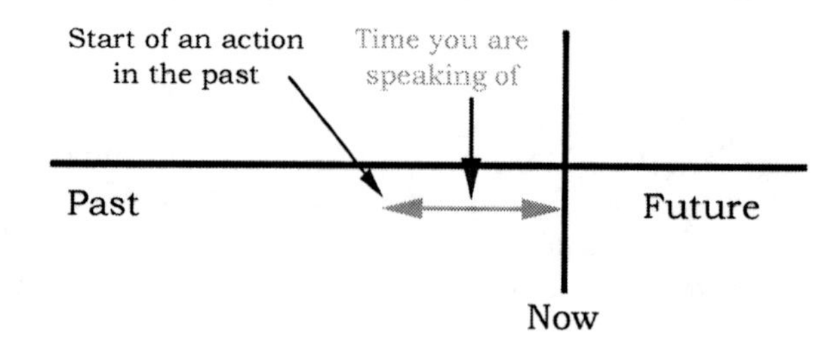

Past Progressive Tense Construction

This tense is formed by using the past tense of the verb "to be" plus the present participle of the main verb.

Sample Question

Bill ________________ lunch when we arrived.

a. will eat
b. is eating
c. eats
d. was eating

How to Answer This Type of Question

1. First examine the question for clues about the time frame.

The sentence ends with "when we arrived," so we know the time frame is a point ("when") in the past (arrived).

The correct answer will refer to an ongoing action at a point of time in the past.

2. Examine the choices and eliminate any obviously incorrect answers.

Choice A is the future tense so we can eliminate.

Choice B is the present continuous so we can eliminate.

Choice C is present tense so we can eliminate.

Choice D refers to an action that takes place at a point of time in the past ("was eating").

2. The Present Perfect Tense

How to Recognize This Tense

I *have had* enough to eat.

We *have been* to Paris many times.

I *have known* him for five years.

I *have been* coming here since I was a child.

About the Present Perfect Tense

This tense expresses the idea that something happened (or didn't happen) at an unspecific time in the past until the present. The action happened at an unspecified time in the past. (If there is a specific time mentioned, the simple past tense is used.) It can be used for repeated action, accomplishments, changes over time and uncompleted action.

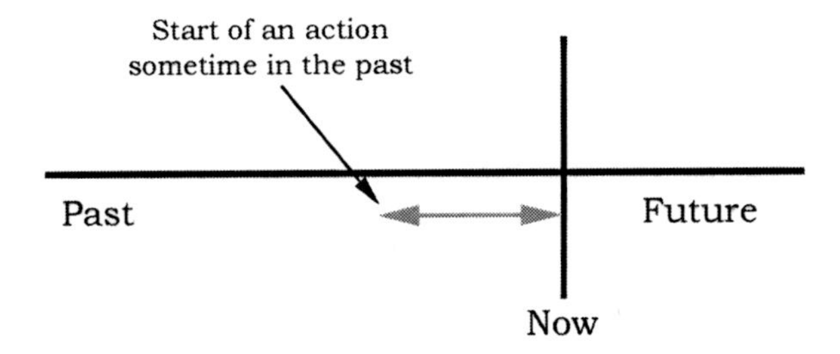

Present Perfect Tense Construction

It is also used with "for" and "since."

This tense is formed by using the present tense of the verb "to have" plus the past participle of the main verb.

Sample Question

I ____________________ these birds many times.

a. am seeing

b. will saw

c. have seen

d. have saw

How to Answer This Type of Question

1. First examine the question for clues about the time frame.

"Many times" tells us that the action is repeated and in the past.

2. Examine the choices and eliminate any obviously incorrect answers.

Choice A, "am seeing" is incorrect because it is a continuing action, i.e. in the present; it also doesn't use a form of 'have'.

Choice B is grammatically incorrect.

Choice C is tells of something that has happened in the past and is now over. Best choice so far.

Choice D is grammatically incorrect.

3. The Present Perfect Progressive Tense

How to Recognize This Tense

We *have been seeing* a lot of rainy days.

I *have been reading* some very good books.

About the Present Perfect Progressive Tense

This tense expresses the idea that something happened (or didn't happen) in the relatively recent past, but the action is not finished. It is used to express the duration of the action.

NOTE: The present perfect speaks of an action that happened sometime in the past, but this action is finished. In the present perfect progressive tense, the action that started in the past is still going on.

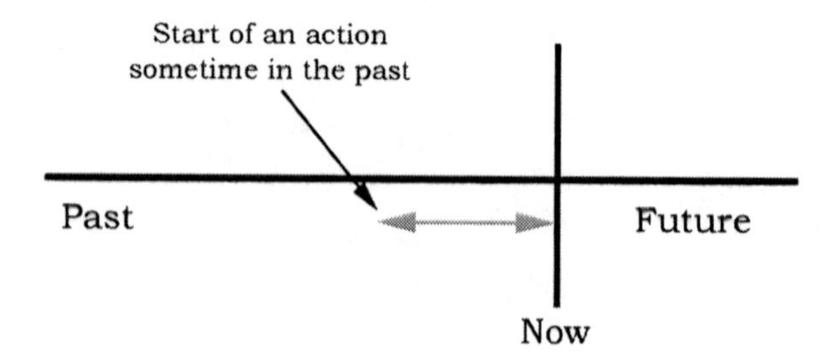

Present Perfect Progressive Tense Construction

This tense is formed by using the present tense of the verb "to have," plus "been," plus the present participle of the main verb.

Sample Question

Bill ____________________ there for two hours.

a. sits

b. sitting

c. has been sitting

d. will sat

How to Answer This Type of Question

1. First examine the question for clues about the time frame.

"For two hours" tells us that the action, "sits," is continuous up to now, and may continue into the future.

Note this sentence could also be the simple past tense,

Bill sat there for two hours.

Or the future tense,

Bill will sit there for two hours.

However, these are not among the options.

2. Examine the choices and eliminate any obviously incorrect answers.

Choice A is incorrect because it is the present tense.
Choice B is incorrect because it is the present continuous. Choice C is correct. "Has been sitting" expresses a continuous action in the past that isn't finished.
Choice D is grammatically incorrect.

4. The Present Progressive Tense

How to Recognize This Tense

We *are having* a delicious lunch.

They *are driving* much too fast.

About the Present Progressive Tense

This tense is used to express what the action is right now. The action started in the recent past, and is continuing into the future.

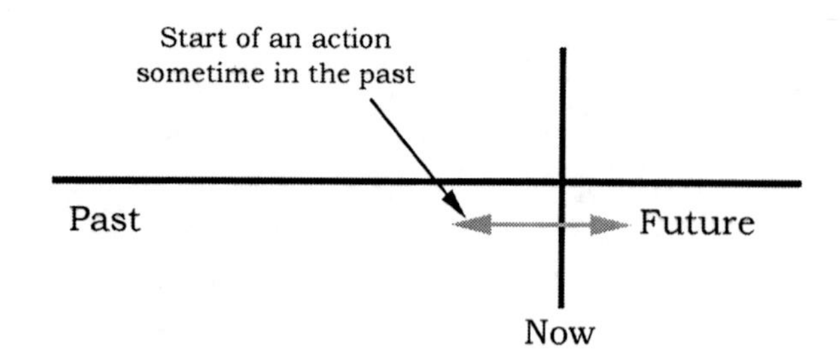

Present Perfect Tense Construction

The Present Progressive Tense is formed by using the present tense of "to be" plus the present participle of the main verb.

Sample Question

She _______________ very hard these days.

a. works

b. is working

c. will work

d. worked

How to Answer This Type of Question

1. First examine the question for clues about the time frame.

The end of the sentence includes "these days" which tell us the action started in the past, continues into the present, and may continue into the future.

2. Examine the choices and eliminate any obviously incorrect answers.

Choice A, the simple present is incorrect.
Choice B, "is working" is correct.
Check the other two choices just to be sure. Choice C is future tense, and Choice D is past tense, so they can be eliminated.

The correct answer is Choice B.

5. The Simple Future Tense

How to Recognize This Tense

I *will see* you tomorrow.
We *will drive* the car.

About the Simple Future Tense

This tense shows that the action will happen some time in the future.

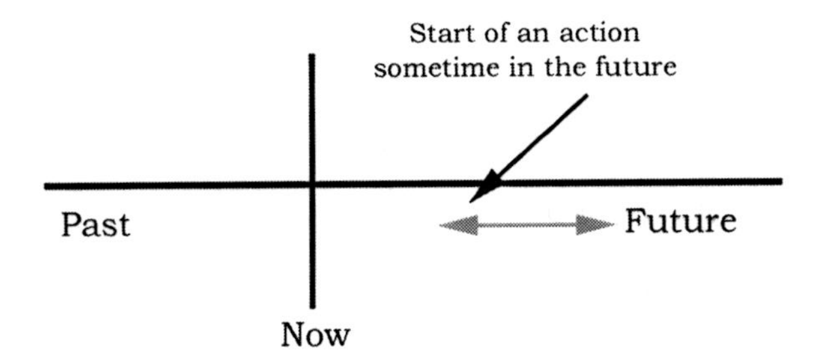

Simple Future Tense Construction

The tense is formed by using "will" plus the root form of the verb. (The root form of the verb is the infinitive without "to." Examples: read, swim.)

Sample Question

We ____________________ to Paris next year.

a. went

b. had been

c. will go

d. go

How to Answer This Type of Question

1. First examine the question for clues about the time frame.

The last two words of the sentence, "next year," clearly identify this sentence as referring to the future.

2. Examine the choices and eliminate any obviously incorrect answers.

Choice A is the past tense and can be eliminated.

Choice B is the past perfect tense and can be eliminated.

Choice D is the simple present and can be eliminated.

Choice C is the only one left and is the correct simple future tense.

6. The Simple Future Tense – The "Going to" Form

How to Recognize This Tense

I *am going to* see you tomorrow.

We *are going to* drive the car.

About the Simple Future Tense

This form of the future tense is used to show the intention of doing something in the future. (This is the strict grammatical meaning, but in daily speech, it is often used interchangeably with the simple future tense, the "will" form.)

The tense is formed by using the present conditional tense of "to go," plus the infinitive of the verb.

Sample Question

I _________________________ shopping in an hour.

a. go

b. have gone

c. am going to go

d. went

How to Answer This Type of Question

1. First examine the question for clues about the time frame.

"In an hour" clearly identifies the action as taking place in the future.

2. Examine the choices and eliminate any obviously incorrect answers.

Choice A is the simple present tense and can also be eliminated.

Choice B is the past perfect and can be eliminated.

Choice C is the correct answer.

Choice D is the past tense and can be eliminated.

7. The Past Perfect Progressive Tense

How to Recognize This Tense

I *had been sleeping* for an hour when you phoned.

We *had been eating* our dinner when they all came into the dining room.

About the Past Perfect Progressive Tense

This tense is used to show that the action had been going on for a period of time in the past when another action, also in the past, occurred.

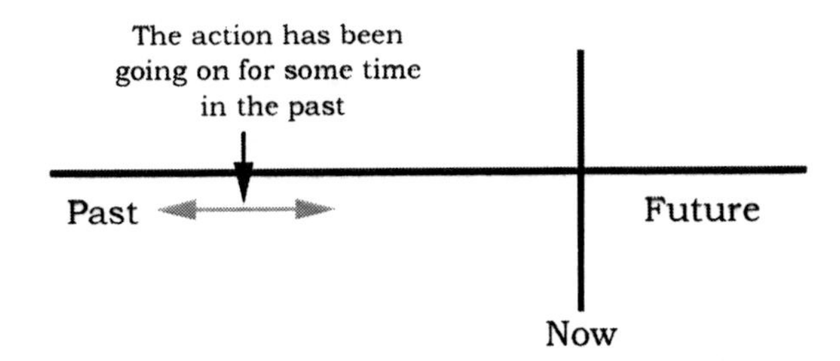

Past Perfect Tense Construction

The tense is formed by using the past perfect tense of the verb "to be" plus the present participle of the main verb.

Sample Question

How long __________ you ____________________ when I saw you?

a. are _____ running
b. had _____ running
c. had _____ been running
d. was _____ running

How to Answer This Type of Question

1. First examine the question for clues about the time frame.

"When I saw" tells us the sentence happened at a point of time ("when") in the past ("saw").

2. Examine the choices and eliminate any obviously incorrect answers.

Choice A, "are running" is incorrect and can be eliminated.

Choice B, “Had ___ running” is grammatically incorrect and can be eliminated.

Choice C is correct.

Choice D is grammatically incorrect so the answer is Choice C.

8. Future Perfect Progressive Tense

How to Recognize This Tense

I *will have been working* here for two years in March.

I *will have been driving* for four hours when I get there, so I will be tired.

About the Future Perfect Progressive Tense

This tense is used to show that the action continues up to a point of time in the future.

Future Prefect Progressive Tense Construction

This tense is formed by using the future perfect tense of “to be” plus the present participle of the main verb.

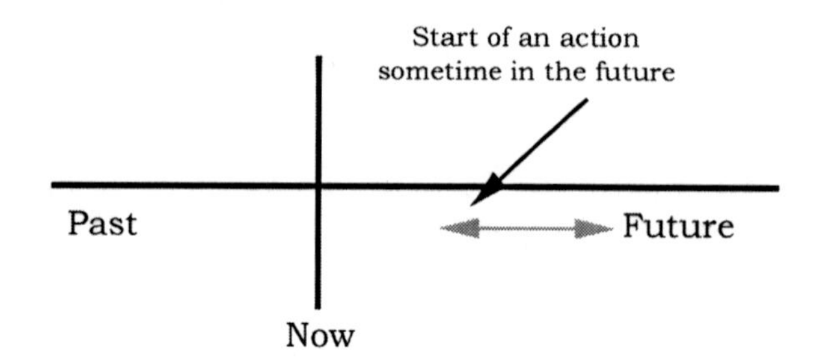

Sample Question

__________ you ______________________________ all the time I am gone?

a. have _____ been working

b. will _____ have been working

c. are _____ worked

d. will _____ worked

How to Answer This Type of Question

1. First examine the question for clues about the time frame.

"All the time I am gone" refers to an action in the future ("time I am gone") and the action is progressive ("all the time"). The progressive action means the correct choice will be a verb tense that ends in "ing."

2. Examine the choices and eliminate any obviously incorrect answers.

Choice A, the past perfect, refers to a past continuous event and is also grammatically incorrect in the sentence, so Choice A can be eliminated.

Choice B looks correct because it refers to an action will be going on for a period of time in the future.

Examine Choices C and D just to be sure. Both choices are grammatically incorrect and can be eliminated.
Choice B is the correct answer.

9. The Future Perfect Tense

How to Recognize This Tense

By next November, I *will have received* my promotion.

By the time he gets home, she is going *to have cleaned* the entire house.

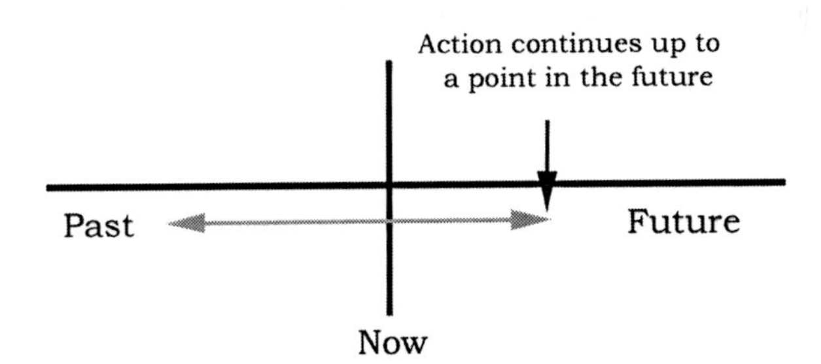

About the Future Perfect Tense

The future perfect tense expresses action in the future before another action in the future. This is the past in the future. For example:

He *will have prepared* dinner when she arrives.

Future Perfect Tense Construction

This tense is formed by "will + have + past participle."

Sample Question

They _____________ their seats before the game begins.

a. will have find

b. will find

c. will have found

d. found

How to Answer This Type of Question

1. First examine the question for clues about the time frame.

This question could be several different tenses. The only clue about the time frame is "before the game begins," which refers to a specific point of time.

We know it isn't in the past, because "begins" is incorrect for the past tense. Similarly with the present. So the question is about something that happens in the future, before another event in the future.

2. Examine the choices and eliminate any obviously incorrect answers.

Choice A can be eliminated as incorrect.
Choice B looks good, so mark it and check the others before making a final decision.
Choice C is the past perfect and can be eliminated because the time frame is incorrect.
Choice D is the simple past tense and can be eliminated for the same reason.

10. Future Progressive Tense

How to Recognize This Tense

The teams *will be playing* soccer when we arrive.

At 3:45 the soccer fans *will be waiting* for the game to start at 4:00 o'clock

At 3:45 the soccer players *will be preparing* to play at 4:00 o'clock

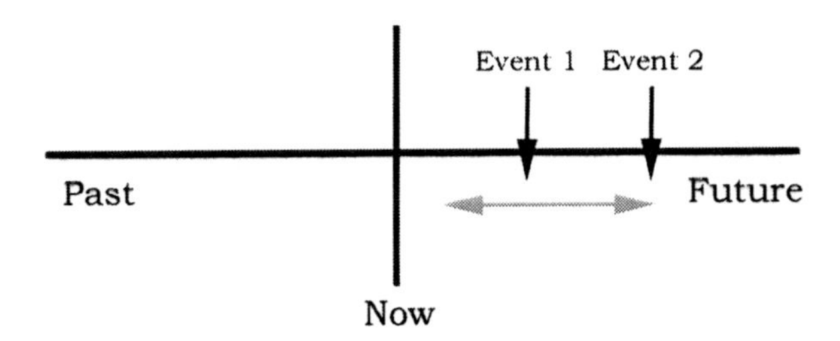

About the Future Progressive Tense

The future progressive tense talks about a continuing action in the future.

Future Progressive Tense Construction

will+ be + (root form) + ing = will be playing

Sample Question

Many excited fans _____________ a bus to see the game at 4:00.

a. catch

b. catching

c. have been catching

d. will be catching

How to Answer This Type of Question

1. First examine the question for clues about the time frame.

"At 4:00," tells us the sentence is either in the past OR in the future.

2. Examine the choices and eliminate any obviously incorrect answers.

From the time frame of the sentence, the answer will be past or future tense.

Choice A is the present tense and can be eliminated.
Choice B is the present continuous tense and can be eliminated.
Choice C is the past perfect continuous and can be eliminated.
Choice D is the only one left. Quickly examining the tense, it is future progressive and is correct in the sentence.

11. The Past Perfect Tense

How to Recognize This Tense

The party *had* just *started* when the coach arrived.

We *had waited* for twenty minutes when the bus finally came.

About the Past Perfect

The past perfect tense talks about two events that happened in the past and establishes which event happened first.

Another example is, “We had eaten when he arrived.”

The two events are “eat” and “he arrived.” From the sentence above the past perfect tense tells us the first event, “eat” happened before the second event, “he arrived.”

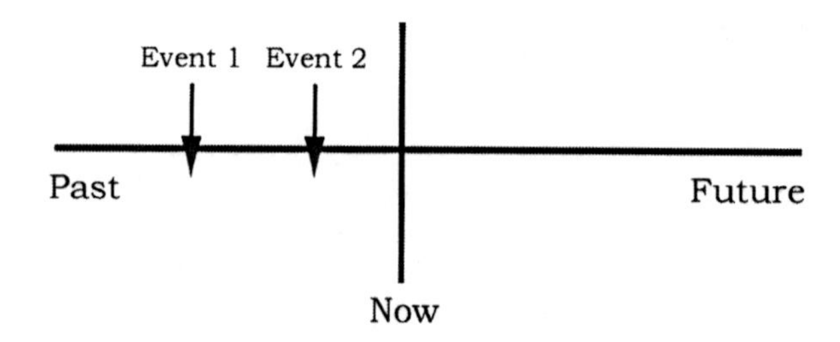

I had already eaten when my friends arrived.

Past Perfect Tense Construction

The past perfect is formed by “have” plus the past participle.

Sample Question

It was time to go home after they __________ the game.

a. will win

b. win

c. had won

d. wins

How to Answer This Type of Question

1. First examine the question for clues about the time frame.

“Was” tells us the sentence happened in the past. Also notice there are two events, “go home” and “after the game.”

2. Examine the choices and eliminate any obviously incorrect answers.

Choice A is the future tense and can be eliminated. Choice B is the simple present and can be eliminated. Choice C is the past perfect and orders the two events in the past. Choice D is the present tense and incorrect and can be eliminated, so Choice C is the correct answer.

Common English Usage Mistakes - A Quick Review

Like some parts of English grammar, usage is definitely going to be on the exam and there isn't any tricky strategies or shortcuts to help you get through this section. Here is a quick review of common usage mistakes.

1. May and Might

'May' can act as a principle verb, which can express permission or possibility.

Examples:

Lets wait, the meeting may have started.
May I begin now?

'May' can act as an auxiliary verb, which an expresses a purpose or wish

Examples:

May you find favour in the sight of your employer.

May your wishes come true.
People go to school so that they may be educated.

The past tense of may is might.

Examples:

I asked if I might begin

'Might' can be used to signify a weak or slim possibility or polite suggestion.

Examples:

You might find him in his office, but I doubt it.
You might offer to help if you want to.

2. Lie and Lay

The verb lay should always take an object. The three forms of the verb lay are: laid, lay and laid.

The verb lie (recline) should not take any object. The three forms of the verb lie are: lay, lie and lain.

Examples:

Lay on the bed.
The tables were laid by the students.
Let the little kid lie.
The patient lay on the table.

The dog has lain there for 30 minutes.

Note: The verb lie can also mean "to tell a falsehood." This verb can appear in three forms: lied, lie, and lied. This is different from the verb lie (recline) mentioned above.

Examples:

The accused is fond of telling lies.
Did she lie?

3. Would and should

The past tense of shall is 'should', and so "should" generally follows the same principles as "shall."

The past tense of will is "would," and so "would" generally follows the same principles as "will."

The two verbs 'would and should' can be correctly used interchangeably to signify obligation. The two verbs also have some unique uses too. Should is used in three persons to signify obligation.

Examples:

I should go after work.
People should do exercises everyday.
You should be generous.

"Would" is specially used in any of the three persons, to signify willingness, determination and habitual action.

Examples:

They would go for a test run every Saturday.
They would not ignore their duties.
She would try to be punctual.

4. Principle and Auxiliary Verbs

Two principle verbs can be used along with one auxiliary verb as long as the auxiliary verb form suits the two principle verbs.

Examples:

A number of people have been employed and some promoted.

A new tree has been planted and the old has been cut down.

Again note the difference in the verb form.

5. Can and Could

A. Can is used to express capacity or ability.

Examples:

I can complete the assignment today
He can meet up with his target.
B. Can is also used to express permission.

Examples:

Yes, you can begin

In the sentence below, "can" was used to mean the same thing as "may." However, the difference is that the word "can" is used for negative or interrogative sentences, while "may" is used in affirmative sentences to express possibility.

Examples:

They may be correct. Positive sentence - use may.
Can this statement be correct? A question using "can."
It cannot be correct. Negative sentence using "can."

The past tense of can is could. It can serve as a principle verb when it is used to express its own meaning.

Examples:

Despite the difficulty of the test, he could still perform well.
"Could" here is used to express ability.

6. Ought

The verb ought should normally be followed by the word to.

Examples:

I *ought to* close shop now.

The verb 'ought' can be used to express:

A. Desirability

You ought to wash your hands before eating. It is desirable to wash your hands.

B. Probability

She ought to be on her way back by now. She is probably on her way.

C. Moral obligation or duty

The government ought to protect the oppressed. It is the government's duty to protect the oppressed.

7. Raise and Rise

Rise
The verb rise means to go up, or to ascend.
The verb rise can appear in three forms, rose, rise, and risen. The verb should not take an object.

Examples:

The bird rose very slowly.
The trees rise above the house.
My aunt has risen in her career.

Raise
The verb raise means to increase, to lift up.
The verb raise can appear in three forms, raised, raise and raised.

Examples:

He raised his hand.
The workers requested a raise.
Do not raise that subject.

8. Past Tense and Past Participle

Pay attention to the proper use these verbs: sing, show, ring, awake, fly, flow, begin, hang and sink.

Mistakes usually occur when using the past participle and past tense of these verbs as they are often mixed up.

Each of these verbs can appear in three forms:

Sing, Sang, Sung.
Show, Showed, Showed/Shown.
Ring, Rang, Rung.
Awake, awoke, awaken
Fly, Flew, Flown.
Flow, Flowed, Flowed.
Begin, Began, Begun.
Hang, Hanged, Hanged (a criminal)
Hang, Hung, Hung (a picture)
Sink, Sank, Sunk.

Examples:

The stranger rang the door bell. (simple past tense)
I have rung the door bell already. (past participle - an action completed in the past)

The stone sank in the river. (simple past tense)
The stone had already sunk. (past participle - an action completed in the past)

The meeting began at 4:00.
The meeting has begun.

9. Shall and Will

When speaking informally, the two can be used interchangeably. In formal writing, they must be used correctly.

“Will” is used in the second or third person, while “shall” is used in the first person. Both verbs are used to express a time or even in the future.

Examples:

I shall, We shall (First Person)
You will (Second Person)
They will (Third Person)

This principle however reverses when the verbs are to be used to express threats, determination, command, willingness, promise or compulsion. In these instances, will is now used in first person and shall in the second and third person.

Examples:

I will be there next week, no matter what.
This is a promise, so the first person “I” takes “will.”

You shall ensure that the work is completed.
This is a command, so the second person “you” takes “shall.”

I will try to make payments as promised.
This is a promise, so the first person “I” takes “will.”

They shall have arrived by the end of the day.
This is a determination, so the third person “they” takes shall.

Note
A. The two verbs, shall and will should not occur twice in the same sentence when the same future is being referred to

Example:

I shall arrive early if my driver is here on time.

B. Will should not be used in the first person when questions are being asked

Examples:

Shall I go ?
Shall we go?

Subject Verb Agreement

Verbs in any sentence must agree with the subject of the sentence both in person and number. Problems usually occur when the verb doesn't correspond to the right subject or the verb fails to match the noun close to it.

Unfortunately, there is no easy way around these principles - no tricky strategy or easy rule. You just have to memorize them.

Here is a quick review:

The verb to be, present (past)

Person	Singular	Plural
First	I am (was)	we are (were)
Second	you are (were)	you are (were)
Third	he, she, it is (was)	they are (were)

The verb to have, present (past)

Person	Singular	Plural
First	I have (had)	we have (had)
Second	you have (had)	you have (had)
Third	he, she, it has (had)	they have (had)

Regular verbs, e.g. to walk, present (past)

Person	Singular	Plural
First	I walk (walked)	we walk (walked)
Second	you walk (walked)	you walk (walked)
Third	he, she, it walks (walked)	they work (walked)

1. Every and Each

When nouns are qualified by "every" or "each," they take a singular verb even if they are joined by 'and'

Examples:

Each mother and daughter *was* a given separate test.
Every teacher and student *was* properly welcomed.

2. Plural Nouns

Nouns like measles, tongs, trousers, riches, scissors etc. are all plural.

Examples:

The trousers *are* dirty.
My scissors *have* gone missing.
The tongs *are* on the table.

3. With and As Well

Two subjects linked by "with" or "as well" should have a verb that matches the first subject.

Examples:

The pencil, with the papers and equipment, *is* on the desk.
David as well as Louis is coming.

4. Plural Nouns

The following nouns take a singular verb:

> politics, mathematics, innings, news, advice, summons, furniture, information, poetry, machinery, vacation, scenery

Examples:

The machinery *is* difficult to assemble
The furniture *has* been delivered
The scenery *was* beautiful

5. Single Entities

A proper noun in plural form that refers to a single entity requires a singular verb. This is a complicated way of saying; some things appear to be plural, but are really singular, or some nouns refer to a collection of things but the collection is really singular.

Examples:

The United Nations Organization *is* the decision maker in the matter.

Here the "United Nations Organization" is really only one "thing" or noun, but is made up of many "nations."

The book, "The Seven Virgins" *was* not available in the library.

Here there is only one book, although the title of the book is plural.

6. Specific Amounts are always singular

A plural noun that refers to a specific amount or quantity that is considered as a whole (dozen, hundred, score etc) requires a singular verb.

Examples:

60 minutes *is* quite a long time.
Here "60 minutes" is considered a whole, and therefore one item (singular noun).

The first million is the most difficult.

7. Either, Neither and Each are always singular

The verb is always singular when used with: either, each, neither, every one and many.

Examples:

Either of the boys *is* lying.
Each of the employees *has* been well compensated
Many a police officer *has* been found to be courageous
Every one of the teachers *is* responsible

8. Linking with Either, Or, and Neither match the second subject

Two subjects linked by “either,” “or,”“nor” or “neither” should have a verb that matches the second subject.

Examples:

Neither David nor Paul *will* be coming.
Either Mary or Tina *is* paying.

Note
If one subject linked by “either,” “or,”“nor” or “neither” is in plural form, then the verb should also be in plural, and the verb should be close to the plural subject.

Examples:
Neither the mother *nor* her kids *have* eaten.
Either Mary *or* her *friends are* paying.

9. Collective Nouns are Plural

Some collective nouns such as poultry, gentry, cattle, vermin etc. are considered plural and require a plural verb.

Examples:

The *poultry are* sick.
The *cattle are* well fed.

Note
Collective nouns involving people can work with both plural and singular verbs.

Examples:

Nigerians are known to be hard working
Europeans live in Africa

10. Nouns that are Singular and Plural

Nouns like deer, sheep, swine, salmon etc. can be singular or plural and require the same verb form.

Examples:

The swine is feeding. (singular)
The swine are feeding. (plural)

The salmon is on the table. (singular)
The salmon are running upstream. (plural)

11. Collective Nouns are Singular

Collective nouns such as Army, Jury, Assembly, Committee, Team etc should carry a singular verb when they subscribe to one idea. If the ideas or views are more than one, then the verb used should be plural.

Examples:

The committee is in agreement in their decision.

The committee were in disagreement in their decision.
The jury has agreed on a verdict.
The jury were unable to agree on a verdict.

12. Subjects links by "and" are plural.

Two subjects linked by "and" always require a plural verb

Examples:

David and John are students.

Note
If the subjects linked by "and" are used as one phrase, or constitute one idea, then the verb must be singular

The color of his socks and shoe is black.
Here "socks and shoe" are two nouns, however the subject is "color" which is singular.

Science

THIS SECTION CONTAINS A SELF-ASSESSMENT AND GENERAL SCIENCE TUTORIALS. The Tutorials are designed to familiarize general principles and the Self-Assessment contains general questions similar to the Science questions likely to be on the DET exam, but are not intended to be identical to the exam questions. Many Universities recommend that students take an introductory science course before taking the DET Exam. The tutorials are not designed to be a complete science course, and it is assumed that students have some familiarity with science. If you do not understand parts of the tutorial, or find the tutorial difficult, it is recommended that you seek out additional instruction.

The Science Self-Assessment covers basic physics, biology, chemistry, physiology and anatomy. The purpose of the self-assessment is:

- Identify your strengths and weaknesses.
- Develop your personalized study plan (above)
- Get accustomed to the DET format
- Extra practice – the self-assessment is a 3rd test!

Since this is a self-assessment, and depending on how confident you are with basic science, timing yourself is optional. There are a total of 75 questions (25 biology, 25 chemistry and 25 Anatomy and Physiology) which must be answered in 75 minutes. The self-assessment has 25 questions, so allow 25 minutes to complete this assessment.

The questions below are not the same as you will find on the DET - that would be too easy! And nobody knows what the questions will be and they change all the time. Below are general Science questions that cover the same areas as the DET. So, while the format and exact wording of the questions may differ slightly, and change from year to year, if you can answer the questions below, you will have no problem with the Science section of the DET.

NOTE: The Science section is an optional module that not all schools include. We strongly suggest that you check with your school for the DET exam details. It is always a good idea to give the materials you receive when you register to take the DET a careful review.

The self-assessment is designed to give you a baseline score in the different areas covered. Here is a brief outline of how your score on the self-assessment relates to your understanding of the material.

75% - 100%	Excellent – you have mastered the content
50 – 75%	Good. You have a working knowledge. Even though you can just pass this section, you may want to review the Tutorials and do some extra practice to see if you can improve your mark.
25% - 50%	Below Average. You do not understand the content. Review the tutorials, and retake this quiz again in a few days, before proceeding to the rest of the practice test questions.
Less than 25%	Poor. You have a very limited understanding. Please review the Tutorials, and retake this quiz again in a few days, before proceeding to the rest of the practice test questions.

Science Self Assessment Answer Sheet

1. (A) (B) (C) (D)
2. (A) (B) (C) (D)
3. (A) (B) (C) (D)
4. (A) (B) (C) (D)
5. (A) (B) (C) (D)
6. (A) (B) (C) (D)
7. (A) (B) (C) (D)
8. (A) (B) (C) (D)
9. (A) (B) (C) (D)
10. (A) (B) (C) (D)
11. (A) (B) (C) (D)
12. (A) (B) (C) (D)
13. (A) (B) (C) (D)
14. (A) (B) (C) (D)
15. (A) (B) (C) (D)
16. (A) (B) (C) (D)
17. (A) (B) (C) (D)
18. (A) (B) (C) (D)
19. (A) (B) (C) (D)
20. (A) (B) (C) (D)
21. (A) (B) (C) (D)
22. (A) (B) (C) (D)
23. (A) (B) (C) (D)
24. (A) (B) (C) (D)
25. (A) (B) (C) (D)

Physics

1. Which of the following is not true of atomic theory?

a. Originated in the early 19th century with the work of John Dalton.

b. Is the field of physics that describes the characteristics and properties of atoms that make up matter.

c. Explains temperature as the momentum of atoms.

d. Explains macroscopic phenomenon through the behavior of microscopic atoms.

2. Which of these statements about atoms is/are incorrect?

a. Are the largest unit of matter that can take part in a chemical reaction.

b. Can be chemically broken down into much simpler forms.

c. Are composed of protons and neutrons in a central nucleus surrounded by electrons.

d. Do not differ in terms of atomic number or atomic mass.

3. Protons, neutrons, and electrons differ in that:

a. Protons and neutrons form the nucleus of an atom, while electrons are found in fixed energy levels around the nucleus of the atom.

b. Protons and neutrons are charged particles and electrons are neutral.

c. Protons and neutrons form fixed energy levels around the nucleus of the atom and electrons are located near the surface of the atom.

d. Protons, neutrons and electrons are charged particles.

4. Which of the statements about quantum theory is/are false?

a. Quantum theory is concerned with the emission and absorption of energy by matter and with the motion of material particles.

b. Quantum mechanics, a system based on quantum theory, has superseded Newtonian mechanics in the interpretation of physical phenomena on the atomic scale.

c. In quantum theory, energy is treated solely as a continuous phenomenon, while matter is assumed to occupy a very specific region of space and to move in a continuous manner.

d. Quantum theory states that energy is held to be emitted and absorbed in tiny, discrete amounts called quantum.

5. Newton's laws of motion consist of three physical laws that form the basis for classical mechanics. Which of the following is/are not included in these laws?

a. Unless acted upon by a force, a body at rest stays at rest.

b. Unless acted upon by a force, a body in motion will change direction and gradually slow until it eventually stops.

c. To every action, there is an equal and opposite reaction.

d. A body acted upon by a force will accelerate in the same direction as the force at a magnitude that is directly proportional to the force.

Biology

6. A ______ ______ is the sequence of developmental stages through which members of a given species must pass.

a. Life cycle

b. Life expectancy

c. Life sequence

d. None of the above

7. Life ________ are the __________ and __________ activities that all ________ systems must be able to carry out in order to maintain life.

a. Life sequences are the chemical and biological activities that all living systems must be able to carry out in order to maintain life.

b. Life expectancies are the biochemical and biophysical activities that all sentient systems must be able to carry out in order to maintain life.

c. Life cycles are the organic and inorganic activities that all living systems must be able to carry out in order to maintain life.

d. Life functions are the biochemical and biophysical activities that all living systems must be able to carry out in order to maintain life.

8. Nutrition is the sum total of activities through which a living organism obtains food; what are the three processes included in nutrition?

a. Ingestion, digestion, and adsorption

b. Ingestion, diffusion, and assimilation

c. Ingestion, digestion, and assimilation

d. Incorporation, digestion, and assimilation

9. _________ is the taking in of food, _________ refers to the chemical changes that take place in the body, and __________ involves the changing of certain nutrients into the protoplasm of cells.

a. Assimilation is the taking in of food, digestion refers to the chemical changes that take place in the body, and ingestion involves the changing of certain nutrients into the protoplasm of cells.

b. Ingestion is the taking in of food, digestion refers to the chemical changes that take place in the body, and assimilation involves the changing of certain nutrients into the protoplasm of cells.

c. Digestion is the taking in of food, ingestion refers to the chemical changes that take place in the body, and assimilation involves the changing of certain nutrients into the protoplasm of cells.

d. Ingestion is the taking in of food, digestion refers to the chemical changes that take place in the body, and diffusion involves the changing of certain nutrients into the protoplasm of cells.

10. The movement of molecules other than water from an area of ____ concentration to an area of _______ concentration is _____.

a. The movement of molecules other than water from an area of high concentration to an area of less concentration is diffusion.

b. The movement of molecules other than water from an area of less concentration to an area of high concentration is diffusion.

c. The movement of molecules other than water from an area of high concentration to an area of less concentration is osmosis.

d. The movement of molecules other than water from an area of lesser concentration to an area of less concentration is dispersal.

11. During _________, a solvent moves through a/an ________ membrane from an area with a_______ concentration of solvents to areas of _______ concentration.

a. During diffusion, a solvent moves through a semipermeable membrane from an area with a lesser concentration of solvents to areas of greater concentration.

b. During osmosis, a solvent moves through an impermeable membrane from an area with a lesser concentration of solvents to areas of greater concentration.

c. During osmosis, a solvent moves through a semipermeable membrane from an area with a greater concentration of solvents to areas of lesser concentration.

d. During osmosis, a solvent moves through a semipermeable membrane from an area with a lesser concentration of solvents to areas of greater concentration.

12. ________ and _______ are forms of ______ transport by which materials pass through plasma membranes.

a. Diffusion and osmosis are forms of active transport by which materials pass through plasma membranes.

b. Diffusion and osmosis are forms of passive transport by which materials pass through plasma membranes.

c. Dispersal and osmosis are forms of passive transport by which materials pass through plasma membranes.

d. Diffusion and synthesis are forms of active transport by which materials pass through plasma membranes.

13. The scientific discipline that studies the physiological aspects, structures, life cycles and division of cells is called _________.

a. The scientific discipline that studies the physiological aspects, structures, life cycles and division of cells is called physiology.

b. The scientific discipline that studies the physiological aspects, structures, life cycles and division of cells is called cell science.

c. The scientific discipline that studies the physiological aspects, structures, life cycles and division of cells is called biochemistry.

d. The scientific discipline that studies the physiological aspects, structures, life cycles and division of cells is called cell biology.

14. Which, if any, of the following statements about mitosis are correct?

a. Mitosis is the process of cell division by which identical daughter cells are produced.

b. Following mitosis, new cells contain less DNA than did the original cells.

c. During mitosis, the chromosome number is doubled.

d. A and C are correct.

15. Which, if any, of the following statements about meiosis are correct?

a. During meiosis, the number of chromosomes in the cell is halved.

b. Meiosis only occurs in eukaryotic cells.

c. Meiosis is the part of the life cycle that involves sexual reproduction.

d. All of these statements are correct.

Chemistry

16. What are the differences, if any, between mixtures and compounds?

a. A mixture is homogeneous, and the properties of its components are retained, while a compound is heterogeneous and its properties are distinct from those of the elements combined in its formation.

b. A mixture is heterogeneous, and the properties of its components are retained, while a compound is homogeneous and its properties are distinct from those of the elements combined in its formation.

c. A mixture is heterogeneous, and the properties of its components are changed, while a compound is homogeneous and its properties are similar to those of the elements combined in its formation.

d. A compound is heterogeneous, and the properties of its components are retained, while a mixture is homogeneous and its properties are distinct from those of the elements combined in its formation.

17. What are the differences, if any, between chemical changes and physical changes?

a. During a physical change, some aspect of the physical properties of matter is altered, but the identity of the substance remains constant. Chemical changes involve the alteration of both a substance's composition and structure.

b. During a chemical change, some aspect of the physical properties of matter is altered, but the identity of the substance remains constant. Physical changes involve the alteration of both a substance's composition and structure.

c. During a physical change, no aspects of the physical properties of matter are altered, but the identity of the substance remains constant. Chemical changes involve the alteration of both a substance's composition and structure.

d. There is no substantive difference between chemical and physical changes.

18. $\Delta H = H_{products} - H_{reactants}$ is the formula used to determine a ______________.

a. Change in hydration

b. Change in haploid bond

c. Change in heat content

d. Change in hypothesis

19. In an ______ reaction, the heat content of the products is ______ than the heat content of the reactants, while in an ________ reaction, the heat content of the products is ______ than the heat content of the reactants.

a. Exothermic, greater, endothermic, less
b. Endothermic, less, exothermic, greater
c. Exothermic, greater, exothermic, less
d. Endothermic, greater, exothermic, less

20. The equation $E = mc^2$ is based on the ________________, and states that ______ equals _____ times the ___________^{2}.

a. The equation $E = mc^2$ is based on the 2nd Law of Thermodynamics, and states that Mass equals Energy times (the Velocity of light) ^{2}.
b. The equation $E = mc^2$ is based on the Law of Conservation of Mass and Energy, and states that Energy equals Mass times (the Velocity of light)^2.
c. The equation $E = mc^2$ is based on the 1st Law of Thermodynamics, and states that Mass equals Energy times (the Velocity of sound) ^{2}.
d. The equation $E = mc^2$ is based on the Law of Conservation of Mass and Energy, and states that the Velocity of light equals Energy times (the Mass)^2.

21. When a measurement is recorded, it includes the ________ ________, which are all the digits that are certain plus one uncertain digit.

a. Major figures
b. Significant figures
c. Relative figures
d. Relevant figures

22. The ______ ______ is based on the lowest theoretical temperature, called ________ _______.

a. Kelvin scale, absolute zero
b. Celsius scale, absolute zero
c. Kelvin scale, boiling point of water
d. Centigrade scale, freezing point of water

23. Through experiments and calculations, _______ _____ has been verified to be ________° on the ________ scale.

a. Through experiments and calculations, absolute zero has been verified to be –273.15° on the Celsius scale.

b. Through experiments and calculations, unconditional zero has been verified to be 0° on the Kelvin scale.

c. Through experiments and calculations, absolute null has been verified to be -100° on the Celsius scale.

d. Through experiments and calculations, absolute zero has been verified to be –273.15° on the Kelvin scale.

24. When using the scientific notation system to express large numbers, move the ______ _____ until ____ digit(s) remain(s) to the left, then indicate the number of moves of the decimal point as the ______ __ ___.

a. When using the scientific notation system to express large numbers, move the decimal point until only two digits remain to the left, then indicate the number of moves of the decimal point as the exponent of 10.

b. When using the scientific notation system to express large numbers, move the decimal until only one digit remains to the left, then indicate the number of moves of the decimal point as the exponent of 2.

c. When using the scientific notation system to express large numbers, move the decimal until only three digits remain to the left, then indicate the number of moves of the decimal point as the exponent of 10.

d. When using the scientific notation system to express large numbers, move the decimal until only one digit remains to the left, then indicate the number of moves of the decimal point as the exponent of 10.

25. In science, _______ indicates the _________ or _________ of a measurement, while ______ indicates the _______ of a measurement to its known or accepted value.

a. In science, accuracy indicates the reliability or reproducibility of a measurement, while precision indicates the proximity of a measurement to its known or accepted value.

b. In science, exactitude indicates the reliability or reproducibility of a measurement, while contiguity indicates the remoteness of a measurement to its known or accepted value.

c. In science, precision indicates the reliability or reproducibility of a measurement, while accuracy indicates the proximity of a measurement to its known or accepted value.

d. In science, uncertainty indicates the realism or possibility of a measurement, while precision indicates the distance of a measurement to its known or accepted value.

Answer Key

1. C
Answer c is incorrect because atomic theory explains temperature as the motion of atoms (faster = hotter), not the momentum. The momentum of atoms explains the outward pressure that they exert.[3]

2. D
The atoms of different elements differ in atomic number, relative atomic mass, and chemical behavior

3. A
Protons and neutrons form the nucleus of an atom, while electrons are found infixed energy levels around the nucleus of the atom.

4. C
In quantum theory, energy is treated solely as a continuous phenomenon, while matter is assumed to occupy a very specific region of space and to move in a continuous manner.

5. B
Unless acted on by a force, a body in motion will change direction and gradually slow until it eventually stops.

This answer is related to Newton's 1st law of motion that states that, unless acted upon by a force, a body at rest stays at rest, and a moving body continues moving at the same speed in a straight line.[4]

Biology

6. A
A **life cycle** is the sequence of developmental stages through which members of a given species must pass.

7. D
Life functions are the biochemical and biophysical activities that all living systems must be able to carry out to maintain life.

8. C
The three processes included in nutrition are, **ingestion, digestion, and assimilation.**

9. C
Ingestion is the taking in of food, **digestion** refers to the chemical changes that take place in the body, and **assimilation** involves the changing of certain nutrients into the protoplasm of cells.

10. A
The movement of molecules other than water from an area of **high** concentration to an area of **less** concentration is **diffusion**.

11. D
During osmosis, a solvent moves through a/an semi permeable membrane from an area with a lesser concentration of solvents to areas of greater concentration.

12. B
Diffusion and **osmosis** are forms of passive transport by which materials pass through plasma membranes.

13. D
The scientific discipline that studies the physiological aspects, structures, life cycles and division of cells is called **cell biology**.

14. A and C are correct.

a. Mitosis is the process of cell division by which a cell produces identical daughter cells.
c. During mitosis, the chromosome number is doubled.

15. D
All these statements are correct.

Chemistry

16. B
A mixture is heterogeneous, and the properties of its components are retained, while a compound is homogeneous and its properties are distinct from those of the elements combined in its formation.

17. A
During a physical change, some aspects of the physical properties of matter are altered, but the identity of the substance remains constant. Chemical changes involve the alteration of both a substance's composition and structure.
Note: Examples of physical changes include breaking glass, cutting wood and melting ice. Sometimes, the process can be easily reversed. Restoration of the original form is not possible following a chemical change.

18. C
ΔH = Hproducts - Hreactants is the formula used to determine a **change in heat content**.

19. D
In an **Endothermic** reaction, the heat content of the products is **greater** than the heat content of the reactants, while in an **exothermic** reaction, the heat content of the prod-

ucts is **less** than the heat content of the reactants.

Because it is virtually impossible to measure the total energy of molecules, the experimental data typically used with reactions is the change in heat content known as enthalpy.

20. B
The equation $E = mc^2$ is based on the **Law of Conservation of Mass and Energy**, and states that **Energy** equals **Mass** times **the Velocity of light**.

21. B
When a measurement is recorded, it includes the **significant figures**, which are all the digits that are certain plus one uncertain digit.

22. A
The Kelvin scale is based on the lowest theoretical temperature, called absolute zero.

23. A
Through experiments and calculations, **absolute zero** has been verified to be **– 273.15°** on the **Celsius** scale.

24. A
When using the scientific notation system to express large numbers, move the **decimal point** until **only two** digits remain to the left, then show the number of moves of the decimal point as the **exponent of 10**.

25. C
In science, **precision** indicates the **reliability** or **reproducibility** of a measurement, while **accuracy** indicates the **proximity** of a measurement to its known or accepted value.

Note: Regardless of the precision or accuracy of a measurement, all measurements include a degree of uncertainty, dependent on limitations of the measuring instrument and the skill with which the measurement is completed.

Science Tutorials

Scientific Method

The scientific method is a set of steps that allow people who ask "how" and "why" questions about the world to go about finding valid answers that accurately reflect reality.

Were it not for the scientific method, people would have no valid method for drawing quantifiable and accurate information about the world.

There are four primary steps to the scientific method:

1. Analyzing an aspect of reality and asking "how" or "why" it works or exists
2. Forming a hypothesis that explains "how" or "why"
3. Making a prediction about the sort of things that would happen if the hypothesis were true
4. Performing an experiment to test your prediction.

These steps vary somewhat depending on the field of science you happen to be studying. (In astronomy, for instance, experiments are generally eschewed in favor of observational evidence confirming that predictions are true.) But for the most part this is the model scientists follow.

Observation and Analysis

The first step in the scientific method requires you to determine what it is about reality that you want to explore.

You might notice that your friends who eat regular servings of fruits and vegetables are healthier and more athletic than your friends who live off red meat and meals covered in cheese and gravy. This is an observation and, noting it, you are likely to ask yourself "why" it seems to be true. At this stage of the scientific method, scientists will often do research to see if anyone else has explored similar observations and analyze what other people's findings have been. This is an important step not only because it can show you what others have found to be true about their observation, but because it can show what others have found to be false, which can be equally as valuable.

Hypothesis

After making your observation and doing some research, you can form your hypothesis. A hypothesis is an idea you formulate based on the evidence you have already gathered about "how" your observation relates to reality.

Using the example of your friends' diets, you may have found research discussing vitamin levels in fruits and vegetables and how certain vitamins will affect a person's health and athleticism. This research may lead you to hypothesize that the foods your healthy friends are eating contain specific types of vitamins, and it is the vitamins making them healthy. Just as importantly, however, is applying research that shows hypotheses that were later proven wrong. Scientists need to know this information, too, as it can help keep them from making errors in their thinking. For instance, you could come across a research paper in which someone hypothesized that the sugars in fruits and vegetables gave people more energy, which then helped them be more athletic. If the paper were to go onto explain that no such link was found, and that the protein and carbohydrates in meat and gravy contained far more energy than the sugar, you would know that this hypothesis was wrong and that there was no need for you to waste time exploring it.

Prediction

The third step in the scientific method is making a prediction based on your hypothesis.

Forming predictions is vital to the scientific method because if your prediction turns out to be correct, it will demonstrate that your hypothesis can accurately explain some aspect of the world. This is important because one aspect of the scientific method is its ability to prove objectively that your way of understanding the world is valid. We can take the simple example of a car that will not start. If you notice the fuel gauge is pointing towards empty, you can announce your prediction to the other passengers that a careful test of the gas tank will show the car has no fuel. While this seems obvious, it is still important to note since a prediction like this is the only way to *prove* to your friends that you understand how a fuel gauge works and what it means.

In the same way, a prediction made by a hypothesis is the only way to show that it represents reality. For instance, based on your vitamin hypothesis you may predict people can be healthy and athletic while eating whatever they want since they take vitamin supplements. If this prediction ends being true, it will show that it is in fact the vitamins, and only the vitamins, in fruits and vegetables that make people healthy and athletic. It will prove that your hypothesis shows how vitamins work.

Experiment

The final step is to perform an experiment that tests your prediction.

You may decide to separate your healthy friends into three groups, give one group vitamin supplements and prohibit them from eating vegetables, give another fake supplements and prohibit them from eating vegetables and have the third act normally as the control group. It is always important to have a control group so you have someone acting "normally" to compare your results against. If this experiment shows the real supplement group and the control group maintaining the same level of health and athleticism while the fake supplement group grows weak and sickly, you will know your hypothesis is true. If, on the other hand, you get unexpected results, you will need to go back to step one, analyze your results, make new observations and try again with a different hypothesis.

Any hypothesis that cannot be confirmed with experiment (or for fields such as astronomy, with observation) cannot be considered true and must be altered or abandoned. It is in this stage where scientists—being humans, with human beliefs and prejudices—are most likely to abandon the scientific method. If an experiment or observation gives a scientist results that he or she does not like, the scientist may be inclined to ignore the results rather than reexamine the hypothesis. This was the case for nearly a thousand years in astronomy with astronomers attempting to form accurate models of the solar system based on circular orbits of the planets and on Earth being in the center. For philosophical reasons many believed that circles were "perfect" and that the Earth was "important," so no model that had the correct elliptical orbits or the sun properly in the center was accepted until the 16th century, even though those models more accurately described all astronomers' observations.

Biology

Biology is a natural science concerned with the study of life and living organisms, including their structure, function, growth, origin, evolution, distribution, and taxonomy.

Biology is a vast subject containing many subdivisions, topics, and disciplines. Among the most important topics are five unifying principles that can be said to be the fundamental axioms of modern biology:

- Cells are the basic unit of life
- New species and inherited traits are the product of evolution
- Genes are the basic unit of heredity
- An organism regulates its internal environment to maintain a stable and constant condition
- Living organisms consume and transform energy.

Sub-disciplines of biology are recognized on the scale at which organisms are studied and the methods used to study them: biochemistry examines the rudimentary chemistry of life; molecular biology studies the complex interactions of systems of biological molecules; cellular biology examines the basic building block of all life, the cell; physiology examines the physical and chemical functions of the tissues, organs, and organ systems of an organism; and ecology examines how various organisms interact and associate with their environment.[5]

Cell Biology

Cell biology (formerly cytology, from the Greek kytos, "contain") is a scientific discipline that studies cells – their physiological properties, their structure, the organelles they contain, interactions with their environment, their life cycle, division and death.

This is done both on a microscopic and molecular level. Cell biology research encompasses both the great diversity of single-celled organisms like bacteria and protozoa, as well as the many specialized cells in multicellular organisms such as humans.

Knowing the components of cells and how cells work is fundamental to all biological sciences.

Appreciating the similarities and differences between cell types is particularly important to the fields of cell and molecular biology as well as to biomedical fields such as cancer research and developmental biology. These fundamental similarities and differences provide a unifying theme, sometimes allowing the principles learned from studying one cell type to be extrapolated and generalized to other cell types. Therefore, research in cell biology is closely related to genetics, biochemistry, molecular biology, immunology, and developmental biology.

Each type of protein is usually sent to a particular part of the cell.

An important part of cell biology is the investigation of molecular mechanisms by which proteins are moved to different places inside cells or secreted from cells.

Processes – Movement of Proteins

Most proteins are synthesized by ribosomes in the rough endoplasmic reticulum.

Ribosomes contain the nucleic acid RNA, which assembles and joins amino acids to make proteins. They can be found alone or in groups within the cytoplasm as well as on the RER.

This process is known as protein biosynthesis.

Biosynthesis (also called biogenesis) is an enzyme-catalyzed process in cells of living organisms by which substrates are converted to more complex products (also simply known as protein translation). Some proteins, such as those to be incorporated in membranes (known as membrane proteins), are transported into the "rough" endoplasmic reticulum (ER) during synthesis. This process can be followed by transportation and processing in the Golgi apparatus.

The Golgi apparatus is a large organelle that processes proteins and prepares them for use both inside, and outside the cell.

The Golgi apparatus is somewhat like a post office. It receives items (proteins from the ER), packages and labels them, and then sends them on to their destinations (to different parts of the cell or to the cell membrane for transport out of the cell). From the Golgi, membrane proteins can move to the plasma membrane, to other sub-cellular compartments, or they can be secreted from the cell.

The ER and Golgi can be thought of as the "membrane protein synthesis compartment" and the "membrane protein processing compartment," respectively.

There is a semi-constant flux of proteins through these compartments. ER and Golgi-resident proteins associate with other proteins but remain in their respective compartments. Other proteins "flow" through the ER and Golgi to the plasma membrane. Motor proteins transport membrane protein-containing vesicles along cytoskeletal tracks to distant parts of cells such as axon terminals.

Some proteins that are made in the cytoplasm contain structural features that target them for transport into mitochondria or the nucleus.

Some mitochondrial proteins are made inside mitochondria and are coded for by mitochondrial DNA. In plants, chloroplasts also make some cell proteins.

Extracellular and cell surface proteins destined to be degraded can move back into intracellular compartments on being incorporated into endocytosed vesicles some of which fuse with lysosomes where the proteins are broken down to their individual amino acids. The degradation of some membrane proteins begins while still at the cell surface when they are separated by secretases. Proteins that function in the cytoplasm are often degraded by proteasomes.

Other cellular processes

Active and Passive transport - Movement of molecules into and out of cells.
Autophagy - The process whereby cells "eat" their own internal components or microbial invaders.
Adhesion - Holding together cells and tissues.

Reproduction - Made possible by the combination of sperm made in the testiculi (contained in some male cells' nuclei) and the egg made in the ovary (contained in the nucleus of a female cell). When the sperm breaks through the hard outer shell of the egg a new cell embryo is formed, which, in humans, grows to full size in 9 months.
Cell movement - Chemotaxis, Contraction, cilia and flagella.
Cell signalling - Regulation of cell behavior by signals from outside.
DNA repair and Cell death
Metabolism - Glycolysis, respiration, Photosynthesis
Transcription and mRNA splicing - gene expression.

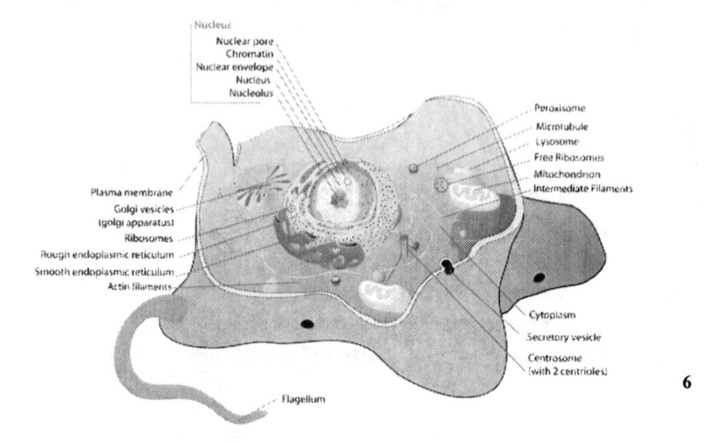

6

Internal cellular structures

Chloroplast - key organelle for photosynthesis (only found in plant cells)
Cilia - motile microtubule-containing structures of eukaryotes
Cytoplasm - contents of the main fluid-filled space inside cells
Cytoskeleton - protein filaments inside cells
Endoplasmic reticulum - major site of membrane protein synthesis
Flagella - motile structures of bacteria, archaea and eukaryotes
Golgi apparatus - site of protein glycosylation in the endomembrane system
Lipid bilayer - fundamental organizational structure of cell membranes
Lysosome - break down cellular waste products and debris into simple compounds (only found in animal cells)
Membrane lipid and protein barrier
Mitochondrion - major energy-producing organelle by releasing it in the form of ATP
Nucleus - holds most of the DNA of eukaryotic cells and controls all cellular activities
Organelle - term used for major subcellular structures
Ribosome - RNA and protein complex required for protein synthesis in cells
Vesicle - small membrane-bounded spheres inside cells

Heredity: Genes and Mutation

All of the genetic material that tells our cells what jobs they hold is stored in our DNA (deoxyribonucleic acid). When complex creatures such as humans reproduce, our DNA is copied and combined with our mate's DNA to create a new genetic sequence for our offspring. This information is stored in our genes and encoded in DNA base pairs through different combinations of the chemical groupings adenine and thymine (represented by A and T) and guanine and cytosine (represented by G and C). Each gene covers a small portion of our DNA and is responsible for creating the protein that section of DNA holds instructions for.

Genes contain two alleles, one from each of our parents. When we reproduce we will transfer one, and only one, of each allele to our children. Alleles can be either dominant or recessive, and by combining the pairs of alleles we get from our parents, we can determine what our genes say we should be like. This genetic description of ourselves is known as our genotype. Genotype is our exact genetic makeup, and it determines our physical characteristics such as basic hair, eye and skin color. Related to the genotype is our phenotype, which describes the characteristics we display when our genes interact with the environment. For example, skin color is determined by a person's genotype, but the effect the sun has on skin—does the person tan, freckle, bun or even come away without any noticeable effect at all?—is an expression of phenotype.

Under normal circumstances people's genes will transfer directly from their parents following Mendel's Laws of Inheritance. DNA reproduction, however, is not necessarily a flawless process. Errors can develop either at random or due to outside influences such as radiation or chemicals in the environment. These errors, when related to heredity are called de novo mutations; they occur during embryonic development. Some mutations have no effect at all on the person's genetic makeup, but others can alter the way genes express themselves. Whether this is a good thing or not depends entirely on what genes are altered in what ways. Some mutations can cause children to be born sick or to have a higher susceptibility to disease by changing the types of proteins that their genes produce, or even by stopping certain proteins from being produced all together. Others, though, can be an improvement to the child's genetic structure. It is important to remember that the entire process of evolution is based on how random mutations throughout history have affected an individual's ability to interact with the environment.

Several notable examples of beneficial mutations stemming from natural selection can be seen in bubonic plague resistant European populations and malaria resistant African populations. Both groups have genes built from specific alleles that create disease blocking proteins. (The CCR5 protein in people of European descent blocks the plague—and HIV sometimes—and the sickle cell protein in people of African descent blocks malaria.) These genes are widespread throughout their respective populations as a result of natural selection, which killed those who lived in these groups' ancestral regions but who did not possess the mutation. Had these diseases never existed, the mutations would have been considered neutral, providing no benefit yet causing no harm.

There are several ways that errors in DNA reproduction can cause mutations. Chemicals can be inserted into, or deleted from base pairs, causing the chemical composition of the pairs to change and, thus, changing the alleles of the gene represented by those pairs. A portion of the DNA strand may also duplicate itself, or it may shift itself, causing the half of the base pair on one side of the DNA strand to link to the wrong half on the other side.

Heredity: Mendelian Inheritance and Punnett Squares

The father of genetics was a 19th century Austrian monk named Gregor Johann Mendel who became famous for his work crossbreeding peas in the garden of his monastery. Aside from his life as a monk, Mendel was a highly educated physicist, studying first at the University of Olomouc (in the modern day Czech Republic) and later at the University of Vienna.

Mendel's work with peas revolutionized the scientific understanding of heredity and yielded two important laws: the Law of Segregation and the Law of Independent Assortment. To better understand these laws, however, we first need to look at the work of another geneticist, Reginald Punnett.

In 1900 while Punnett was doing his graduate work at the University of Cambridge in England, Gregor Mendel's work on genetics, which did not receive much attention during his lifetime, was being rediscovered. Punnett became an early follower of Mendelian genetics and developed the Punnett square as a means to organize the assortment of inherited alleles as Mendel described them. A Punnett square is simply a box with several squares drawn inside it and with the allele for a particular gene from each parent listed on either the top or the side. Each square shows a possible genotype (or set of alleles that define the gene) that can be inherited by the offspring of those parents. We will see Punnett squares as we explain Mendel's laws.

Law of Segregation

Mendel's Law of Segregation says that only half of the alleles of each parent's genes are transferred to their offspring, with the other half coming from the other parent. Each gene contains two alleles. For instance a gene for trait 'A' could contain the alleles AA, Aa or aa, with the 'A' being the dominant form of the allele and 'a' being the recessive form. (Offspring with one or more dominant alleles exhibit the trait; offspring with only recessive forms do not.) The Law of Segregation says that one allele will come from one parent, and one will come from the other, and it is the parent's combined genetic make-up (rather than one parents particular genotype) that will determine the genes of their offspring.

Mendel also showed that the probability a certain trait would spread from parents to children was 3:1, if both parents had one dominant and one recessive form of the gene, also known as having heterozygous alleles. (Having two of the same alleles—AA or aa—is homozygous.) To get a better understanding of this, we can use a Punnett square to demonstrate the process.

The Punnett square below represents the possible children born to two parents with Aa alleles expressing the 'A' gene.

	A	a
A	**AA**	**Aa**
a	**Aa**	aa

The three genes in bold, with at least one capital letter (AA, Aa and the other Aa), represent cases in which the presence of at least one dominant allele will cause the trait to manifest in the offspring. The remaining one (aa) represents the one case where the child does not manifest the trait even though both his or her parents do. (This could be the one brunette in a family of redheads, for instance.) Provided both parents have one dominant and one recessive allele, the distribution will always be 3:1.

Law of Independent Assortment

Mendel's second law, the Law of Independent Assortment, shows that the alleles of multiple genes will mix independently of each other. When two separate genotypes are tracked, the genes will produce 16 separate possible combinations spread out in a 9:3:3:1 ratio. This is also known as a dihybrid cross, while dealing with a single set of alleles is a monohybrid cross.

We can demonstrate this by assuming that we have a male and a female each with heterozygous alleles making them blond and tall. We can represent this with the genotypes BbTt in each. We should also assume that a 'bb' genotype would give someone brown hair and 'tt' would make them short. Since the Law of Independent Assortment says that each allele will mix independently, we end with four combinations of genotype that each parent can pass on: BT, Bt, bT and bt. These can then be mapped in a slightly larger Punnett square that looks like this:

	BT	Bt	bT	bt
BT	***BBTT***	***BBTt***	***BbTT***	***BbTt***
Bt	***BBTt***	**BBtt**	***BbTt***	**Bbtt**
bT	***BbTT***	***BbTt***	*bbTT*	*bbTt*
bt	***BbTt***	**Bbtt**	*bbTt*	bbtt

This is the distribution of the tall, blond couple's possible children. Nine would also be tall and blond, three would be short and blond, three would be tall and brunette, and one would be short and brunette. This perfectly follows the 9:3:3:1 ratio set out by Mendel.

Classification

Classification

Taxonomic classification is the primary method of organizing the Earth's biology. Taxonomy means,

> **1. The classification of organisms in an ordered system that indicates natural relationships.**
> **2. The science, laws, or principles of classification**

The earliest form of classification that bears any resemblance to the current system can be traced back to ancient Greece with Aristotle's organization of animals based on reproduction.

The classification into kingdoms (animal, mineral and vegetable) was developed by Carolus Linnaeus.

> The true father of modern taxonomical classification, however, is Carolus Linnaeus, who in the early 18th century developed a system of kingdoms that separated life into the categories animal, mineral and vegetable. Although Linnaeus's work lacked what would today be considered essential technologies (such as microscopes capable of imaging bacteria) and theories (such as evolution), much of his system has survived in modern classification.

Charles Darwin's theory of evolution was an important factor in taxonomic classification.

> With Charles Darwin's publication of On the Origin of Species in 1859 the evolutionary process became a major factor in taxonomic classification. For the first time biology could be classified by grouping the direct descendents of common ancestors rather than just grouping creatures with similar characteristics.

The main classifications are, domain, kingdom, phylum, class, order, family, genus and species.

> Today, most scientists accept a hierarchical structuring of biology that goes from general, or large, to specific: domain, kingdom, phylum, class, order, family, genus and species. (There are sometimes smaller subcategories such as superfamily, subfamily, tribe and subspecies listed, but these are the primary eight categories.) Domain is the newest of these and is split into three primary groups: Bacteria, Archaea and Eukarya.
>
> Each of these domains is split again with Bacteria splitting into the Kingdom Bacteria, Archaea splitting into the Kingdom Archaea and Eukarya splitting into the four kingdoms of Protista, Plantae, Fungi and finally our kingdom, Animalia. The Domain Eukarya splits so many times because eukaryotic cells

are highly complex, containing such important features as cell walls and nuclei. As a result of this complexity, eukaryotic cells have gone through a much more diverse evolutionary process than prokaryotic cells such as bacteria and archaea, and thus Eukarya make up all complex life on Earth

Rank	**Fruit fly**	**Human**	**Pea**	***E. coli***
Domain	Eukarya	Eukarya	Eukarya	Bacteria
Kingdom	Animalia	Animalia	Plantae	Bacteria
Phylum or **Division**	Arthropoda	Chordata	Magnoliophyta	Proteobacteria
Subphylum or subdivision	Hexapoda	Vertebrata		
Class	Insecta	Mammalia	Magnoliopsida	
Subclass	Pterygota	Theria	Rosidae	
Order	Diptera	Primates	Fabales	
Suborder	Brachycera		Fabineae	
Family	Drosophilidae	Hominidae	Fabaceae	
Subfamily	Drosophilinae	Homininae	Faboideae	
Genus	*Drosophila*	*Homo*	*Pisum*	*Escherichia*
Species	*D. melanogaster*	*H. sapiens*	*P. sativum*	*E. coli*

7

Each Kingdom has a huge number of organisms. Bacteria and Archaea (single celled organisms).

Within each of the kingdoms the number of creatures is far too many to list. It is estimated that there could be as many as 100 million different species on Earth, although nowhere near that many have been physically catalogued. Of these, the majority are Bacteria and Archaea.

Another Example - Homo Sapiens

Since there is no way to list all the different subdivisions of life on Earth here, we might as well focus on one specific animal: us, Homo sapiens. We are members of the Domain Eukarya, the Kingdom Animalia, the Phylum Chordata, the Class Mammalia, the Order Primates, the Family Hominidae, the Genus Homo, the Species Homo sapiens and finally the Subspecies Homo sapiens sapiens. This classification is able to demonstrate our exact biological position relative to life on Earth.

One important thing that a system like this tells us is that Homo, which is Latin for "human," is not actually our species, but our genus. This is an easy fact to forget since we are currently the only member of our genus not yet extinct. But anthropologically speaking there have been many humans including Homo habilis, Homo erectus and Homo neanderthalensis.

Taxonomical classification is an evolutionary map

Furthermore, the taxonomical classification system can be seen as a map of evolution on the planet. Plants, animals and bacteria can be traced back to common ancestors and newly discovered species can be classified relative to their ancestors, descendants and cousins. The Genus Homo, for instance, is a direct offshoot of the Tribe Hominini. (A tribe is a subcategory of the category of family, which here is Hominidae.) Another genus that falls under the Tribe Hominini is Pan, which houses the species Chimpanzee. This shows us that until relatively recently in the history of life, Homo sapiens and Chimpanzees were the same creature, and that Chimpanzees only split off just before Homo sapiens became fully human.

Ecology

Ecology is the scientific study of the relationship between the Earth and its life forms. The purpose of ecology is to understand the structures that occur in nature.

Ecologists study the planet's ecosystems, the various communities of living things (biotic) and non-living structures (abiotic) that occur in localized areas throughout the world. The purpose of ecology is to understand the organizational structures that occur spontaneously in nature. Within an ecosystem there are different levels of organization which are broken down by relative size. Each ecosystem is composed of communities of animals, and within each community exist numerous populations, or individual species groups.

Ecosystems Ecology

Ecosystems ecology studies areas that can be differentiated from neighboring areas by the types of rocks, soil and other non-living features, as well as the types of plants and animals adapted to live there.

A desert ecosystem may boarder an arid grassland ecosystem, which in turn may boarder a forest ecosystem. The purpose of ecosystems ecology is to analyze the system of interactions the animals and plants in a particular area have with the non-living portions environment. It also focuses heavily on local evolution, studying what traits are favored within particular ecosystems and why.

Ecosystems can be qualified.

Many quantifiable factors go into making an ecosystem. Abiotic components are things such average sunlight, temperature, average rainfall and moisture levels, soil composition and other similar factors. Similarly, biotic components consist of the number and type of primary producers (generally plants), secondary producers (herbivores) and tertiary producers (carnivores and omnivores). All of this information can be quantified. For example, ecologists can calculate the amount of energy in a system by studying average amount of sunlight, the efficiency of photosynthesis in local plants, calories that exist in prey animals, nutrients absorbed by bacteria from breaking down dead predators and so on. Provided all of the factors have been accounted for, this sort of quantitative analysis of ecosystems can help ecologists determine factors such as the efficiency of the food web and the maximum supportable population. It can also help determine accurate ways to repair damaged ecosystems.

Community Ecology

Community ecology looks at similar regions to ecosystems ecology but focuses primarily on the biotic factors, ignoring the abiotic.
In ecological terms a community describes the interactions of several species in a local area. Ecologists define these interactions between species in several ways: mutualism, interaction where both species benefit such as between bees and flowering plants; commensalism, interaction where one species benefits and the other neither notices nor minds; competition, interaction where both species are harmed; and predation or parasitism, interaction where one species is benefitted while the other is harmed such as predators attacking prey or herbivores eating plants.

A local food web, is a graphical representation showing who eats what in nature.

To ecologists, however, food webs are much more specific, showing the transfer of energy from organism to organism. Energy moves from lower trophic levels to higher ones. Trophic levels are the various positions that plants and animals occupy within the food web relative to other plants and animals that they want to eat or that want to eat them. Plants, for instance, would have a lower trophic level than grazing animals such as deer. Similarly, deer would have lower trophic levels than wolves.

Within communities species can be affected by changes either directly (such as when they are eaten by their main predator) or indirectly (such as when their main predator has its numbers diminished by a new and even bigger predator). There are also cascading effects on communities, such as when a dominant herbivorous species dies out and all its former prey (both plant and animal) increase drastically in number.

Each organism occupies a trophic level (or position) in the food chain.

A food chain represents a succession of organisms that eat another organism and are, in turn, eaten themselves. The number of steps an organism is from the start of the chain is a measure of its trophic level. The simplest is the first trophic level (level 1) is plants, then herbivores (level 2), and then carnivores (level 3).

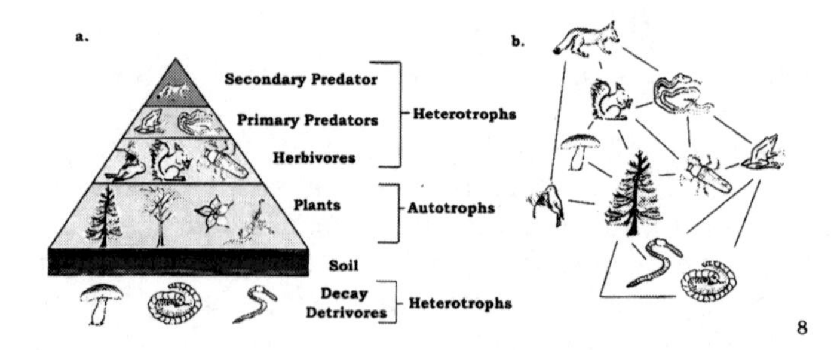

A trophic pyramid (a) and a simplified community food web (b) illustrating ecological relations among creatures that are typical of a northern Boreal terrestrial ecosystem. The trophic pyramid roughly represents the biomass (usually measured as total dry-weight) at each level. Plants generally have the greatest biomass. Names of trophic categories are shown to the right of the pyramid. Some ecosystems, such as many wetlands, do not organize as a strict pyramid, because aquatic plants are not as productive as long-lived terrestrial plants such as trees. Ecological trophic pyramids are typically one of three kinds: 1) pyramid of numbers, 2) pyramid of biomass, or 3) pyramid of energy

Population Ecology

Population Ecology studies a single species and the primary factor is population size.

Getting even more specific is population ecology, which focuses on only one species either within a community or across a large space. The primary characteristic of a population is its size. Population sizes can change due to an imbalance in the number of births and deaths as well as plants and animals emigrating to new areas.

Ecologists who study populations will generally model their growth rates to make predictions about the species. One method is the exponential growth model, which looks at current population trends and, assuming that they will remain constant, shows the increase or decrease in population over numerous generations. The other method is the logistic growth model, which slows reproduction when populations reach a certain density and increases it when they drop below a certain density to account for the increase in predators and decrease in the food supply that often follows massive population growth.

Natural Selection and Adaptation

Natural selection and adaptation are one of the fundamental teachings of evolution. Natural selection is the non-random gradual process that biological traits become more common or less common among a population.

The theory of natural selection was made popular by Charles Darwin and was first introduced in his 1859 book; The Origin of Species.

As species and organisms evolve, some mutations and changes in the genomes occur as they interact with their environments. These changes and mutations can be passed from the organism to its offspring. In time, individual organisms or living beings with particular traits or genome variants may survive and produce offspring more successfully than individuals with different traits or genome variants. As this process goes on, the population slowly evolves as individuals with weak traits relative to their environment die out or are replaced by individuals with the right traits or mutations to survive. This is why the process of natural selection is also sometimes called the survival of fittest.

Over time as species and organisms continue to react to their environment and develop traits and genome variants to suit their environment they may become specialized to suit a particular environment niche, and new species may even be produced. Natural selection is thus an important pillar of evolution although it is not the only process that leads to evolution.

Natural selection differs with artificial selection because the latter involves the purposeful selection of specific favorable traits by humans.

With natural selection, the individual organism doesn't make the choice, but the changing environment determines which traits are necessary for survival and individual organisms that lack the required traits would die out.

Not all variants and mutations affect the survival of the individual.

For example, the difference in eye color among a population such as among humans is not necessarily a survival factor. However, a rabbit that develops the trait of running faster and passes it onto its offspring does have improved chances of escape and survival from predators than rabbits that do not. The same would be true for algae that successfully develop the trait or ability to extract more energy from sunlight, such algae would outgrow others without this trait.

Adaptation

Adaptation is a process in which an organism evolves to be better able to live and survive in its habitat or environments.

Adaptation is closely related to natural selection and it covers both the state of being adapted to the environment and the process that led to the adaptation. Adaptation is also a fundamental teaching of evolution as popularized by Charles Darwin.

Organisms existing in their various environments face several challenges that they must adapt to survive. An organism must develop observable phenotype

traits in response to the conditions imposed on it by its environment for it to survive and thrive.

The ability of an organism to adapt is thus closely linked to its fitness and survival. Adaptation is not exactly simple or fast. It may take a period of small steps for the entire process to be complete and for the organism to be fully adapted. During all the stages of adaptation and evolution, the organism has to be viable to be able to survive the process.

Adaptation is a process in which the phenotype of the organism changes to better suit the environment. There are many classical examples of adaptation. An animal that develops thick fur to survive the cold environment has adapted, just as the case of an animal that develops effective camouflage techniques to hide itself from predators.

Adaptation can be behavioral, structural or physiological.

Structural adaptation has to do with changes in physical features such as body covering, physical defense mechanism, size and shape and some internal restructuring.

Physiological adaptations allow the organism to do perform unique functions such as secreting slime, making venom or phototropism. Physiological adaptations include general functions such as temperature regulation, development and growth and ionic balance.

Behavioral adaptations include inherited behaviors and mannerisms as well as the ability to learn. Inherited behaviors are termed instinct and may include mating style, food search and vocalizations.

Chemistry

Chemistry is the science of matter, especially its chemical reactions, but also its composition, structure and properties. Chemistry is concerned with atoms and their interactions with other atoms, and particularly with the properties of chemical bonds.

Chemistry is sometimes called "the central science" because it connects physics with other natural sciences such as geology and biology. Chemistry is a branch of physical science but distinct from physics.

Traditional chemistry starts with the study of elementary particles, atoms, molecules, substances, metals, crystals and other aggregates of matter. in solid, liquid, and gas states, whether in isolation or combination. The interactions, reactions and transformations that are studied in chemistry are a result of interaction either between different chemical substances or between matter and energy.

A chemical reaction is a transformation of some substances into one or more other substances.

It can be symbolically depicted through a chemical equation. The number of atoms on the left and the right in the equation for a chemical transformation is most often equal. The nature of chemical reactions a substance may undergo and the energy changes that may accompany it are constrained by certain basic rules, known as chemical laws.

Energy and entropy considerations are invariably important in almost all chemical studies.

Chemical substances are classified in terms of their structure, phase as well as their chemical compositions. They can be analyzed using the tools of chemical analysis, e.g. spectroscopy and chromatography. Scientists engaged in chemical research are known as chemists. Most chemists specialize in one or more subdisciplines. [7]

Basic Concepts in Chemistry

Atoms

Atoms are some of the basic building blocks of matter. Each atom is an element—an identifiable substance that cannot be further broken down into other identifiable substances.

There are just over 100 such elements, and each of them can combine with themselves and with other elements to create all the various molecules that exist in the universe. The poison gas chlorine and the explosive metal sodium, for instance, can combine at the atomic level to form sodium chloride, also known as salt.

For thousands of years atoms were thought to be the smallest thing possible. (The word “atom” comes from an ancient Greek word meaning “unbreakable.”) However, experiments performed in the mid to late 19th century began to show the presence of small particles, electrons, in electric current. By the early 20th century, the electron was known to be a part of the atom that orbited a yet undefined atomic core. A few years later, in 1919, the proton was discovered and found to exist in the nuclei of all atoms.

The protons and neutrons inside an atomic nucleus are not fundamental particles. That is, they can be divided into still smaller pieces.

Protons and neutrons are known as hadrons, which is a class of particle made up of quarks. (Quarks are a fundamental particle.) There are two distinct types of hadrons, baryons and mesons, and both protons and neutrons are baryons, meaning they are both made up of a combination of three quarks. In addition to being hadrons, protons and neutrons are also known as nucleons because of their place within the nucleus. Protons have a mass of around 1.6726 × 10−27 kg and neutrons have a nearly identical mass of 1.6929 × 10−27 kg. Both particles have a ½ spin.

The number of protons inside an atomic nucleus determines what element the atom is.

An element with only one proton, for instance, is hydrogen. An element with two is helium. One with three is lithium, and so on. No element (except for hydrogen) can exist with only protons in its nucleus. Atoms need neutrons to bond the protons together using the strong force. In general atoms (again except for hydrogen) have an equal number of protons and neutrons in their nuclei.

Atoms with an uneven number of protons and neutrons are called isotopes.

Isotopes have all the same chemical properties as their evenly balanced counterparts, but their nuclei are not usually as stable and are more willing to react with other elements. (Two deuterium atoms, hydrogen isotopes with one proton and one neutron in their nucleus rather than only one proton, will fuse much more readily than two regular hydrogen atoms.)

Nearly all an atoms' mass is within its nucleus. Outside that, there is empty space occupied only by a few, tiny electrons.

Electrons were once viewed as orbiting an atom like planets orbit the sun. We now know that this is wrong in several ways. For one, electrons do not really "orbit" in the sense we are used to. At the quantum level no particle is really a particle, but is actually both a particle and a wave simultaneously. Heisenberg's uncertainty principle looks at this odd truth about reality and says that never can you watch an electron orbit the nucleus as you would watch the Earth orbit the sun. Instead, you have to observe only one of the electron's physical characteristics at a time, either viewing it as a particle in a fixed position outside the nucleus or as a wave encircling the nucleus like a halo.

Additionally, planets orbiting their stars can orbit at any distance they want. In fact, every object in our solar system has an elliptical orbit, meaning that they all move in more oval rather than circular shapes, getting closer and farther from the sun at various points. Electrons cannot do this under any circumstances.

Atoms have what are known as electron shells, which are the levels that an electron is able to occupy.

Electrons cannot exist in between these shells; instead they jump from one to the next instantaneously. Each electron shell can hold a different number of atoms. When a shell fills up, additional electrons fill the outer shells. The outermost shell of any atom is called the valence shell, and it is the electrons in this shell that interact with the electrons of other atoms. The important thing about the valence shell is that each electron shell has a specific number of electrons that it can hold, and it wants to hold that many.

When atoms join; their connecting valence electrons take up two valence shell spots, one on each atom.

This means that the fewer electrons an atom has in its valence shell, the more likely it is to interact with other atoms. Conversely, the more electrons it has, the less likely it is to interact.

Electrons can also momentarily jump from one electron shell to the next if they are hit with a burst of energy from a photon.

When photons hit atoms, the energy is briefly absorbed by the electrons, and this momentarily knocks them into higher "orbits." The particular "orbit" the electron is knocked into depends on the type of atom, and when the electron gives up its higher energy level it re-emits a photon at a slightly different wavelength than the one it absorbed, providing a characteristic signal of that atom and showing exactly what "orbit" the electron was knocked into.

This is the phenomenon responsible for spectral lines in light and is the reason we can tell what elements make up stars and planets just by looking at them.

Unlike protons and neutrons, electrons are a fundamental particle, all on their own. They are known as leptons.

Electrons have a negative charge that is generally balanced out by the positive charge of their atom's protons.

Charged atoms, which have either gained or lost an electron for various reasons, are called ions.

Ions, like isotopes, have the same properties that the regular element does; they simply have different tendencies towards reacting with other atoms. Electrons have a mass of 9.1094 × 10-31 kg and a -½ spin.

Element

The concept of chemical element is related to that of chemical substance. A chemical element is specifically a substance which is composed of a single type of atom.

A chemical element is characterized by a particular number of protons in the nuclei of its atoms. This number is known as the atomic number of the element. For example, all atoms with 6 protons in their nuclei are atoms of the chemical element carbon, and all atoms with 92 protons in their nuclei are atoms of the element uranium.

Compound

A compound is a substance with a particular ratio of atoms of particular chemical elements which determines its composition, and a particular organization which determines chemical properties.

For example, water is a compound containing hydrogen and oxygen in the ratio of two to one, with the oxygen atom between the two hydrogen atoms, and an angle of 104.5° between them. Compounds are formed and interconverted by chemical reactions.

Substance

A chemical substance is a kind of matter with a definite composition and set of properties.

Strictly speaking, a mixture of compounds, elements or compounds and elements is not a chemical substance, but it may be called a chemical. Most of the substances we encounter in our daily life are some kind of mixture; for example: air, alloys, biomass, etc.

Nomenclature of substances is a critical part of the language of chemistry. Generally it refers to a system for naming chemical compounds.

Earlier in the history of chemistry substances were given names by their discoverer, which often led to some confusion and difficulty. However, today the IUPAC system of chemical nomenclature allows chemists to specify by name specific compounds amongst the vast variety of possible chemicals.

The standard nomenclature of chemical substances is set by the International Union of Pure and Applied Chemistry (IUPAC). There are well-defined systems in place for naming chemical species. Organic compounds are named according to the organic nomenclature system. Inorganic compounds are named according to the inorganic nomenclature system. In addition the Chemical Abstracts Service has devised a method to index chemical substance. In this scheme each chemical substance is identifiable by a number known as CAS registry number.

Molecule

Molecules are two or more atoms joined together through a chemical bond to form chemicals.

Molecules differ from atoms in that molecules can be further broken down into smaller pieces and into elements while atoms cannot. (This was actually the 18th century definition of an atom: a recognizable structure that could no longer be broken down into smaller bits.)

Atoms are joined into molecules in two main ways: through covalent bonds and through ionic bonds.

Covalent bonds are the primary type of chemical bond that forms molecules. They occur when atoms with only partially filled valence electron shells, an atom's outermost electron shell, come together to share electrons. Hydrogen atoms, for instance, each have only one electron, while their valence shell is capable of holding two. When two hydrogen atoms come together each share the other's electron, using it to occupy its valence shell's free space forming the H2 molecule: hydrogen gas.

Not all covalent bond's are the same.

Different atoms have different levels of positive charge coming from in their nuclei, and although, under normal circumstances, the negative charge of the atom's electrons balances that out (keeping the atom electrically neutral) the chemical bonding process has a way of exploiting this situation. If we look at the H2 molecule again, everyday experience tells us that it has a strong tendency to seek out and bond with oxygen (O) molecules forming H20, or water. There are two main reasons for this. The first comes from the regular old covalent bonds that are already holding H2 together. If bonded to another atom, hydrogen gains the ability to form a new valence shell that can hold 6 electrons. Since oxygen is the only molecule to naturally have 6 electrons in its valence shell, it is the most eager to bond with hydrogen. However, oxygen also has 8 protons in its nucleus compared to the total of 2 in the H2 molecule. This means that as the atoms come closer and prepare to bond, the electrons from both atoms are pulled closer to the oxygen molecule and farther from the hydrogen. An atom's proclivity to pull electrons towards itself is called its electronegativity, and this process creates polar covalent bonds. Due to this connection, polar covalent bonds are the strongest molecular bond, which is why molecules like water are so prevalent in our solar system and, likely, throughout the galaxy.

One very interesting aspect of polar covalent bonds is the hydrogen bond.

When a hydrogen atom bonds with another electronegative atom, the newly created molecule develops an intense polar attraction to all other electronegative atoms. This attraction works almost like a magnet with one end of the molecule exhibiting a positive charge (due to the effects of the polar covalent bonds pulling all the electrons towards one end of the molecule) and the other end exhibiting a negative charge. This phenomenon is responsible for, among other things, the way water molecules stick to each other so readily. This is why you can fill a glass of water to a millimeter or so above the rim before it spills.

Hydrogen bonds are also responsible for how hydrophilic and hydrophobic molecules react to being mixed with water.

Hydrophilic molecules are molecules like NaCl (salt) which exhibit their own strong charge for reasons we will discuss in a moment. The charged salt molecules mix eagerly with the charged water molecules due to the extra pull of the hydrogen bond. Conversely, hydrophobic molecules such as oil will not mix with water because they are neutrally charged and do not like charged molecules. This is the reason you have to shake up an oil based salad dressing each time you use it. The oil and the water never truly mix, and given only a short amount of time they will separate.

A very different type of bond between atoms is called the ionic bond.

Ionic bonds only occur between ions, atoms that are either positively or negatively charged due to having an unequal number of protons and electrons. Ionic bonds always occur between metals and non-metals, such as the gas chlorine (Cl) and the alkaline metal sodium (Na). In their normal states, neither of these elements are ions, but when they approach each other, the sodium gives the chlorine one of its electrons forming Cl^- and Na^+ ions, which subsequently become attracted to one another. Since no electrons are actually lost, the molecule still technically has a neutral charge; it is only the atoms that are charged.
In ionic bonds it is always the metal which gives its electron to the non-metal. Additionally, in a diluted or liquid form, molecules that are created like this will always conduct electricity. This is why salt water can make such a good conductor.

Ions and salts

An ion is a charged species, an atom or a molecule, that has lost or gained one or more electrons.

Positively charged cations (e.g. sodium cation Na^+) and negatively charged anions (e.g. chloride Cl^-) can form a crystalline lattice of neutral salts (e.g. sodium chloride NaCl). Examples of polyatomic ions that do not split up during acid-base reactions are hydroxide (OH^-) and phosphate (PO_4^{3-}).

Ions in the gaseous phase are often known as plasma.

Acidity and basicity

A substance can often be classified as an acid or a base. There are several different theories which explain acid-base behavior. The simplest is Arrhenius theory.

The Arrhenius theory states than an acid is a substance that produces hydronium ions when it is dissolved in water, and a base is one that produces hydroxide ions when dissolved in water. According to Brønsted–Lowry acid-base theory, acids are substances that donate a positive hydrogen ion to another substance in a chemical reaction; by extension, a base is the substance which receives that hydrogen ion.

A third common theory is Lewis acid-base theory, which is based on the formation of new chemical bonds.

Lewis theory explains that an acid is a substance which is capable of accepting a pair of electrons from another substance during the process of bond formation, while a base is a substance which can provide a pair of electrons to form a new bond. According to concept as per Lewis, the crucial things being exchanged are charges. There are several other ways in which a substance may be classified as an acid or a base, as is evident in the history of this concept

Acid strength is commonly measured by two methods. The most common is pH.

One measurement, based on the Arrhenius definition of acidity, is pH, which is a measurement of the hydronium ion concentration in a solution, as expressed on a negative logarithmic scale. Thus, solutions that have a low pH have a high hydronium ion concentration, and can be said to be more acidic. The other measurement, based on the Brønsted–Lowry definition, is the acid dissociation constant (Ka), which measure the relative ability of a substance to act as an acid under the Brønsted–Lowry definition of an acid. That is, substances with a higher Ka are more likely to donate hydrogen ions in chemical reactions than those with lower Ka values.

Phase

Besides the specific chemical properties that distinguish chemical classifications, chemicals can exist in several phases.

For the most part, the chemical classifications are independent of these bulk phase classifications; however, some more exotic phases are incompatible with certain chemical properties. A phase is a set of states of a chemical system that have similar bulk structural properties, over a range of conditions, such as pressure or temperature.

Physical properties, such as density and refractive index tend to fall within values characteristic of the phase. The phase of matter is defined by the phase transition, which is when energy put into, or taken out of the system goes into rearranging the structure of the system, instead of changing the bulk conditions.

Phase can be continuous.

Sometimes the distinction between phases can be continuous instead of having a discrete boundary, here the matter is considered to be in a supercritical state. When three states meet based on the conditions, it is known as a triple point and since this is invariant, it is a convenient way to define a set of conditions.

The most familiar examples of phases are solids, liquids, and gases. Many substances exhibit multiple solid phases. For example, there are three phases of solid iron (alpha, gamma, and delta) that vary based on temperature and pressure. A principle difference between solid phases is the crystal structure, or arrangement, of the atoms. Another phase commonly encountered in the study of chemistry is the aqueous phase, which is the state of substances dissolved in aqueous solution (that is, in water).

Less familiar phases include plasmas, Bose-Einstein condensates and fermionic condensates and the paramagnetic and ferromagnetic phases of magnetic materials. While most familiar phases deal with three-dimensional systems, it is also possible to define analogs in two-dimensional systems, which has received attention for its relevance to systems in biology.[9]

Redox

Redox is a concept related to the ability of atoms of various substances to lose or gain electrons.

Substances that can oxidize other substances are said to be oxidative and are known as oxidizing agents, oxidants or oxidizers. An oxidant removes electrons from another substance. Similarly, substances that can reduce other substances are said to be reductive and are known as reducing agents, reductants, or reducers.

A reductant transfers electrons to another substance, and is thus oxidized itself. And because it "donates" electrons it is also called an electron donor.

Oxidation and reduction properly refer to a change in oxidation number—the actual transfer of electrons may never occur. Thus, oxidation is better defined as an increase in oxidation number, and reduction as a decrease in oxidation number.

Bonding

Electron atomic and molecular orbitals

Atoms sticking together in molecules or crystals are said to be bonded with one another.

A chemical bond may be visualized as the multipole balance between the positive charges in the nuclei and the negative charges oscillating about them. More than simple attraction and repulsion, the energies and distributions characterize the availability of an electron to bond to another atom.

A chemical bond can be a covalent bond, an ionic bond, a hydrogen bond or just because of Van der Waals force.

Each of these kinds of bond is ascribed to some potential. These potentials create the interactions which hold atoms together in molecules or crystals. In many simple compounds, Valence Bond Theory, the Valence Shell Electron Pair Repulsion model (VSEPR), and the concept of oxidation number explains molecular structure and composition.

Reaction

During chemical reactions, bonds between atoms break and form, resulting in different substances with different properties.

In a blast furnace, iron oxide, a compound, reacts with carbon monoxide to form iron, one of the chemical elements, and carbon dioxide.

When a chemical substance is transformed as a result of its interaction with another or energy, a chemical reaction is said to have occurred. Chemical reaction is therefore a concept related to the 'reaction' of a substance when it comes in close contact with another, whether as a mixture or a solution; exposure to some form of energy, or, both. It results in some energy exchange between the constituents of the reaction as well with the system environment which may be designed vessels which are often laboratory glassware.

Chemical reactions can result in the formation or dissociation of molecules, that is, molecules breaking apart to form two or more smaller molecules, or rearrangement of atoms within or across molecules.

Chemical reactions usually involve the making or breaking of chemical bonds. Oxidation, reduction, dissociation, acid-base neutralization and molecular rearrangement are some of the commonly used kinds of chemical reactions.

A chemical reaction can be symbolically depicted through a chemical equation. While in a non-nuclear chemical reaction the number and kind of atoms on both sides of the equation are equal, for a nuclear reaction this holds true only for the nuclear particles viz. protons and neutrons.

The sequence of steps in which the reorganization of chemical bonds may be taking place in the course of a chemical reaction is called its mechanism.

A chemical reaction can be envisioned to take place in several steps, each of which may have a different speed. Many reaction intermediates with variable stability can thus be envisaged during a reaction. Reaction mechanisms are proposed to explain the kinetics and the relative product mix of a reaction. Many physical chemists specialize in exploring and proposing the mechanisms of various chemical reactions. Several empirical rules, like the Woodward-Hoffmann rules often come handy while proposing a mechanism for a chemical reaction.

Equilibrium

Although the concept of equilibrium is widely used across sciences, in the context of chemistry, it arises whenever several different states of the chemical composition are possible.

For example, in a mixture of several chemical compounds that can react with one another, or, when a substance can be present in more than one kind of phase.

A system of chemical substances at equilibrium even though having an unchanging composition is most often not static; molecules of the substances continue to react, causing a dynamic equilibrium. Thus the concept describes the state in which the parameters such as chemical composition remain unchanged over time. Chemicals present in biological systems are invariably not at equilibrium; but are far from equilibrium.

The Periodic Table

The periodic table contains the known chemical elements displayed in a special tabular arrangement based on their electron configurations, atomic numbers and recurring chemical properties.

The first semblance of a periodic table was by Antoine Lavoisier in 1789. He published a list or table of the 33 chemical elements known since then. He grouped the elements into earths, non-metals, gases and metals. The next century after that discovery saw several chemists looking for a better classification method and this caused the periodic table as we have it today.

Structure of the Periodic Table

The standard periodic table as it is today is an 18 column by 7 rows table containing the main chemical elements. Beneath that is a smaller 15 column by 2 rows table. The periodic table can be broken down into 4 rectangular blocks: the P block is by the right, S block is left, D block is at the middle and the F block is underneath that. The elements in the blocks are based on which sub-shell the last electron resides.

The chemical elements on the table are arranged in order of increasing atomic number, which refers to the number of protons of the element. The periodic table can be used to study the chemical behavior of chemical elements, which makes it a very important tool widely used in chemistry.

The periodic table contains only chemical elements. Mixtures, compounds or small atomic particles of elements are not included. Each element on the table has a unique atomic number, which represents the number of protons contained in the element's nucleus.

A new period or row begins when an element has a new electron shell with a first electron. Columns or groups are based on the configuration of electrons of the atom. Elements that have an equal number of atoms in a specific sub-shell are listed under the same column. For example, selenium and oxygen both have 4 electrons in their outermost sub shell and so are listed under the P column. Elements with similar properties are listed in the same group although some elements in the same period can also share similar properties too. Since the elements grouped together have related properties, one can easily predict the property of an element if the properties of the surrounding elements are already known.

Rows are Periods

The rows of the periodic table are called periods. Elements on a row have the same number of electron shells or atomic orbitals. Elements on the first row have just one atomic orbital, elements on the second row have 2, and so it goes until the elements on the seventh row that have 7 electron shells or atomic orbitals.

Columns are Groups

Columns from up to down in the table are called groups. The columns in the D, P and S blocks are called groups. Elements within a group have equal number of electrons in their outermost electron shell or orbital. The electrons on the outer shell are called valence electrons and there are the electrons that combine with other elements in a chemical reaction.

The Periodic table contains natural and synthesized elements

The elements up to californium are natural existing elements (94) while the rest were laboratory synthesized. Chemists are still working to produce elements beyond the present 118th element, ununoctium. 114 of the 118 elements on the table have been officially recognized by the International Union of Pure and Applied Chemistry (IUPAC). Elements listed on the table under 113, 115, 117 and 118 have been synthesized but are yet to officially recognized by the IUPAC and are only known by their systematic element names.

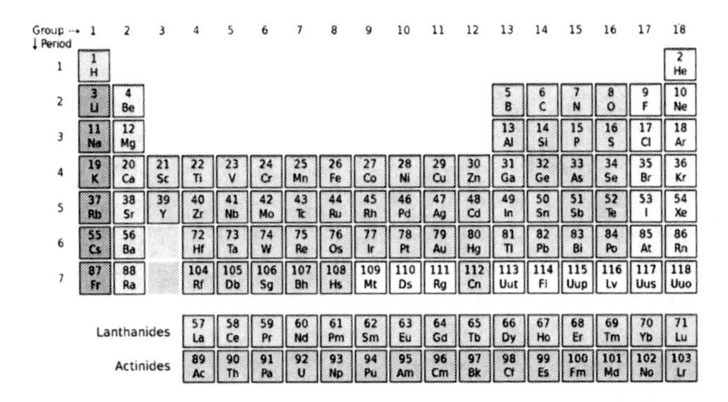

Chemistry and Energy

In the context of chemistry, energy is an attribute of a substance because its atomic, molecular or aggregate structure. Since a chemical transformation is accompanied by a change in one or more of these kinds of structure, it is invariably accompanied by an increase or decrease of energy of the substances involved.

Some energy is transferred between the surroundings and the reactants of the reaction as heat or light; thus the products of a reaction may have more or less energy than the reactants.

Exergonic, Endergonic, Exothermic and Endothermic

A reaction is said to be exergonic if the final state is lower on the energy scale than the initial state; for endergonic reactions the situation is the reverse. A reaction is said to be exothermic if the reaction releases heat to the surroundings;

for endothermic reactions, the reaction absorbs heat from the surroundings.

Chemical reactions are invariably not possible unless the reactants surmount an energy barrier known as the activation energy.

The speed of a chemical reaction (at given temperature T) is related to the activation energy E, by the Boltzmann's population factor e – E / kT - that is the probability of molecule to have energy greater than or equal to E at the given temperature T. This exponential dependence of a reaction rate on temperature is known as the Arrhenius equation. The activation energy necessary for a chemical reaction can be as heat, light, electricity or mechanical force in sound.

Basic Physics

Kinetic and Mechanical Energy

The kinetic energy of an object is the energy it possesses due to its motion.

Kinetic energy is the work needed to accelerate a body of a given mass from rest to a stated velocity. Like all forms of energy, kinetic energy is measured in joules. Kinetic energy can be imparted to an object when an energy source is tapped to accelerate it. It can also happen when one object with kinetic energy slams into another object and kinetic energy from the first object is transferred to the second.

However it happens, imparting kinetic energy to an object causes it to accelerate. In this way movement is nothing more than an indication of the quantity of kinetic energy an object has. An object will hold onto its kinetic energy until it is able to transfer it to something else, which allows it to slow down again.

As long as an object has the same level of kinetic energy, it will move at a consistent velocity forever. This is Newton's first law of motion.

The transfer of kinetic energy from one object to another can occur in many ways.

The transfer of kinetic energy can be as simple and mundane as a baseball flying through the air—interacting with all the various molecules of oxygen, carbon dioxide, nitrogen and all the other gasses that make up our atmosphere, and transferring its kinetic energy to them—speeding them up and slowing itself down in the process. Or it can be as chaotic as a speeding truck losing control on an icy road and slamming into a wall.

Different types of interactions between objects appear to be different but are in fact the same.

The interaction between the baseball and the air and between the truck and the wall are only superficially different. One appears more chaotic than the other only because of the differences in mass between a baseball and a truck and the differences in "negative energy" possessed by free-floating air molecules compared to a solid wall. At its most basic, however, the same events are taking place in both examples. Molecules in both the wall and the air scatter when the kinetic energy they receive, causes them to move, and this causes both heat and sound to be produced.

Kinetic energy can be calculated with the formula $KE=\frac{1}{2}mv^2$ where m is the mass of the object in kilograms, and v is its velocity in meters/second.

Kinetic energy increases by the square of an objects velocity.

One important aspect of kinetic energy that makes it so potentially destructive is that the kinetic energy a moving object carries does not increase on pace with its velocity, but relative to the square of its velocity. If you double an object's velocity, you will quadruple the quantity of kinetic energy it possesses (22=4). If you quadruple the velocity, you increase the kinetic energy by sixteen times (42=16). This can lead to relatively small masses possessing very high kinetic energy levels when they are accelerated to only nominally high speeds. This is one reason why modern kinetic energy weapons (such as firearms) are able to cause large amounts of damage while being extremely compact.

Mechanical Energy

Mechanical energy is the ability of an object to do work.

When discussing energy it is important to take a moment to understand mechanical energy and how it relates to the objects it interacts with. Mechanical energy is not a separate type of energy in the way that potential energy and kinetic energy differ from each other.

Mechanical energy is the potential energy available to an object added to all of the kinetic energy available to it, providing a total energy output.

For instance, in our description of potential energy there is the example of a pole-vaulter hanging in mid air with her pole bent at a near right angle to the ground. The bend in the pole-vaulter's pole contains elastic potential energy, which will help her clear the bar. However, that is not the only source of energy the pole-vaulter is restricted to. For anyone who has ever seen a track and field competition, you know that pole-vaulters take long, running starts before planting their poles in the ground. This imparts kinetic energy to the runners body, and it is that kinetic energy plus the pole's elastic potential energy that are added together in mid air to impart the total mechanical energy that drives the pole-vaulter high into the air and over the bar.

Potential Energy

There are two main types of potential energy: gravitational potential energy and elastic potential energy.

Potential energy is quite simply the potential an object has to act on other objects. As gravitational potential energy, the object is raised off the ground and is waiting for the force of gravity pulling at $9.8m/s^2$, to grab hold of it and pull it towards the Earth.

This type of energy is very common in everyday life. It describes everything from a book falling off its shelf to a child tripping on a crack in the sidewalk. Because gravitational potential energy is so common, the equation describing it PEgrav=mass*g*height should not be hard to figure out since it contains only easily observable features of matter: an object's mass, the force of gravity (g), and the object's height off the ground when it started falling.

Note that the height does not have to be measured from the ground. Any point can be chosen—such as a table top or even a point in mid-air—provided that you are only concerned with the energy an object would have if it fell from the point it was currently at to the point you have chosen.

Gravitational Potential Energy Example

If we take the example of a 1kg weight positioned at a height of 1 meter above the surface of Earth (where the gravity is $9.8m/s^2$—try this on Mars and you will get a different result), we end with the equation PEgrav=1*9.8*1, which equals 9.8 joules of gravitational potential energy. A 1g weight positioned at the same height would be PEgrav=.001*9.8*1 or, 0098J of potential energy, while a 1kg weight positioned a kilometer up would equal PEgrav=1*9.8*1000 or 9800J of potential energy.

From this equation you may have picked up on the fact that the height an object is raised to is directly proportional to the amount of gravitational potential energy it has. Take a 1kg object and raise it to 5m, and you get 49J of potential energy. Double that to 10m, and you get 98J. Triple it to 15m and you will get 147J—three times the original 49J.

Elastic Potential Energy

Elastic potential energy occurs when an object is stretched or compressed out of its normal "resting" shape. The quantity of energy that will be released when it finally returns to rest is the quantity of elastic potential energy it has while stretched or compressed.

A common example of elastic potential energy is when an archer draws back the string of his bow. The farther back the bowstring is pulled, the more it will stretch. The more it stretches the more potential energy that it will have waiting to send into the arrow.

Elastic potential energy of an object can be determined using Hooke's law of elasticity. Hooke's law states that F=-kx where F is the force the material will exert as it returns to its resting state measured in Newtons, x is the amount of displacement the material undergoes measured in meters, and k is the spring constant and is measured in Newtons/meter.

To determine the potential energy of an elastic or springy material you use the equation $PE=\frac{1}{2}kx^2$. According to this equation, an object such as a spring with a spring constant of 5N/m that is stretched 3 meters past its resting point would have a potential energy of 22.5J. That is, ½*5*32 = 2.5*9 = 22.5J.

Remember that elastic potential energy affects much more than just what you would consider elastic or springy material such as rubber bands, bungee cords and springs. There is elastic potential energy in a pole-vaulter's pole at the point where she is in the air and hanging onto a pole that is bent nearly sideways. In the next instant her forward momentum will be boosted by the conversion of her pole's potential energy into kinetic energy, pushing her over the bar. Similarly, when a hockey player shoots the puck, he drags his stick along the ice as it moves forward, bending the shaft backwards slightly. This adds extra force to the puck as the stick snaps forward back into its normal resting position.

Energy: Work and Power

In the simplest terms, energy is the ability to do work.

Energy allows objects and people to affect the physical world and displace (or move) other objects or people.

Work in the physics sense is a very specific concept.

It is measured in joules, which are 1 Newton of force that displaces something by 1 meter. (J=Nm) As the mass of the object being displaced varies, the quantity of work in joules required to move it a meter will vary too.

To determine the amount of work being done, you can use the equation W=F*d*cosΘ.

This defines work as the force applied, multiplied by the distance the object was displaced, multiplied by the cosine of Θ (Theta).

The force is measured in Newtons. Distance is measured in meters. The tricky part of this equation is determining the cosine of Θ. Θ represents the difference in angle between the vector (or direction) the force is acting in and the vector the displacement is occurring. That means that there are really only three possible values for Θ.

If the force is pushing or pulling in one direction, and the object being displaced is moving in that same direction, then there is no difference in angle between the vectors and $\Theta=0°$. This is the sort of force you get when a child pulls her sled across a snowy field. The direction the child is pulling and the direction the sled is traveling are the same. Since $\cos 0=1$ the quantity of work is determined by multiplying the force and the displacement.

You should note that the angle of the vectors is determined by their relationship to each other and not to some ideal flat surface. That is, if the child is pulling her sled up a steep hill rather than across a field, the angle of Θ is still going to be 0° since the force she exerts on the sled and the sled itself are still traveling in the same direction.

The second possibility is when the force vector acts in the opposite direction of the object's displacement. This gives you what is called "negative work" because the energy is working to hinder the object from moving rather than to help it. In this instance $\Theta=180°$ since the vector in which the force is acting and the vector in which the object is moving are opposite. This force is most commonly observed when dealing with friction. It is the reason that hockey pucks and soccer balls will not travel forever; the force of friction exerted by the ice and by the grass is acting in the opposite direction.

The final difference in vectors is when the force being exerted on an object is at a right angle to its displacement. Here $\Theta=90°$. You can picture this as a waitress carrying a tray of drinks over to your table, and it provides for some odd conclusions. Since the force we are talking about is the force the waitress is using to hold the tray vertically, but the displacement vector of the tray is horizontally across the room, we find that the force the waitress exerts does no work at all. It is not responsible for moving the tray horizontally towards your table.

This is represented mathematically with the fact that the $\cos 90=0$, meaning that the original equation $W=F*d*\cos\Theta$ would be $W=F*d*0$. Without adding any other information in, it is already obvious that work is going to equal zero joules.

A different way to imagine this is to think of cargo in the back of a truck.

It took work to load the cargo up onto the truck from the ground (the force vector and the displacement vector were both pointing in the same direction), but once the cargo was loaded, no additional work was required to keep it there. The truck could drive from one end of the country to the other, but zero joules of work would be exerted keeping the cargo in place in the back of the truck.

When you add a unit of time to your calculations of work, you get a new classification: power.

Power is the rate at which work is done. The equation that measures power is power=work/time. In this equation work is measured in joules, time is measured in seconds and power is measured in watts.

Since, as we noted above, one joule is the same as one Newton multiplied by one meter, this equation can also be written as power=(force*displacement)/ time where force is measured in Newtons and displacement is measured in meters. However, this opens up further possibilities. Since the math does not care whether we first multiply force with displacement before dividing the whole thing by time, or whether we divide displacement by time and then multiply the answer by force, we find the equation can also be written as power=force(displacement/time).

Given that displacement is measured in meters and the time in seconds, what we are really saying here is that power equals the amount of force applied to an object multiplied by that object's velocity (m/s).

Thus we get two equations describing power: power=work/time and power=force*velocity.

By definition, power has an inverse relationship with time; the less time it takes for the work to be done, the more power is being applied. Power also has a direct relationship with force and velocity. Increase either the quantity of force being applied to an object, or the speed at which it is traveling, and you have increased the power.

Defining Force and Newton's Three Laws

In physics force is the term given to anything that has the power to act on an object, causing its displacement in one direction or another.

Forces are an abstract concept, and it is therefore that it took thousands of years to identify accurately and describe them. It was not until the 17th century when a man named Isaac Newton began to describe accurately the basic physical forces and show how they acted on matter.

Force is measured using the unit Newton (N). One Newton can be defined with the formula $1N=1kg(1m/s^2)$. In other words, if you accelerate a kilogram of matter by one meter per second per second, you have exerted one Newton of force on it.

Newton developed three laws to explain the interactions of matter he observed. The first is often known as the "Law of Inertia."

It states that an object at rest will stay at rest, and an object in motion will stay in motion, unless a force acts on it to change its state. This means that if you fire a spaceship out into the vacuum of space, and keep it clear from planets and stars that will apply force to it, the ship will keep going at the same speed forever.

This tendency to stay moving or stay at rest is known as inertia. Inertia is directly related to an object's mass; the more mass an object has, the more inertia it will have and the harder that it will be to speed it up or slow it down. The equation implies this, defining one Newton of force, but it is also obvious in everyday life. You have to exert more force to push a box of books across the floor than you would to push a box of clothes the same size. The box of books has more mass, so it has more inertia. Similarly, a baseball player can easily catch and stop a baseball thrown at over 100km/hr. If you were to ask that same player to stop a truck traveling at 100km/hr, you would get much less pleasant results.

One important thing to remember about force is that it is a vector quantity, meaning that it points in a specific direction.

Set a one kilogram object down on a table and you will have the force of gravity pulling it down at one Newton, and the force of all the atoms in the table pushing it up at one Newton. This is said to be a state of equilibrium, and it causes no change to the object's velocity. However, if the table had been poorly built and was only capable of pushing up at .75 Newtons, the object would pull through, snapping the table at its weakest points, and fall until it found something that was capable of applying the needed force to hold it up against gravity.

As such, an object can only be at rest if it has no forces acting on it, or if it has equal and opposite forces acting on it keeping it at equilibrium. If an unopposed force acts on an object, it will move.

Newton's second law deals with what happens when you have the sort of unbalanced forces that we just described.

It explains the movement of objects through the equation $F=ma$, where F is the force in Newtons, m is the object's mass in kilograms, and a is the object's acceleration in meters per second per second (m/s2).

Just like with Newton's first law, this equation shows that mass is a huge player when it comes to using a force to move objects. The larger the mass, the more force you will need to accelerate or decelerate it to the same velocity.

Newton's third law states simply that for every action there is an equal and opposite reaction.

This means that if I pound my hand down on my desk right now, my desk will also be hitting up at my hand with the exact same force. This may sound strange, but it is the reason that pounding your hand on your desk can damage your desk and hurt your hand at the same time. It is also the reason that baseball bats can snap while imparting force onto the ball, and why a moving car hitting stationary wall will damage both.

Force: Friction

Friction is the force that resists the motion of objects relative to other objects.

When two surfaces move relative to each other, the force of friction is what slows them down. Friction applies to all matter, whether it is a book sliding down a slanting shelf, a soccer ball rolling on the ground or a baseball flying though the air. Friction is a constant opposing force that keeps things from traveling forever.

Several laws describe how friction works.

Amontons' first law of friction says that, "The force of friction is directly proportional to the applied load." His second law of friction says that, "The force of friction is independent of the apparent area of contact." Similarly, Coulomb's law of friction states that, "Kinetic friction is independent of the sliding velocity."

The two main types of Friction are static friction and kinetic friction.

Static friction is what you get when one stationary object is stacked on top of another stationary object, such as a book resting on a table. The static friction between the book and the table determines how much sticking power there is between them, and at what angle you would have to tilt the table before the force of gravity overpowers the force of friction and starts the book sliding. To figure out the maximum amount of static friction possible before the book starts sliding, you use the formula $f s = \mu s F n$ where $f s$ is the total amount of static friction, μs (pronounced "mu") is the coefficient of static friction and Fn is the "normal force," the force being exerted perpendicularly through the surface into the object resting on it, keeping the object from breaking through the surface.

Another way to examine static friction is to calculate the angle the table will have to reach before the book will start sliding.

This is also known as the angle of repose, and it can be calculated using the formula $\tan\theta = \mu s$ where θ (pronounced "theta") is the angle of repose and μs is the coefficient of static friction.

Aside from determining the angels that books will slide off tables, calculating static friction allows tire manufacturers to determine how "grippy" their treads are. If there were no friction, the wheel would not be a functional tool because it would not push itself against the road while moving. The higher the coefficient of friction between the tire and the road, the more grip the tire has.

Kinetic friction is sort of the inverse of static friction.

It is the force that causes moving objects to slow down. Kinetic friction applies to two surfaces moving in respect to one another such as the bottom of a snowboard and the snowy ground. It can be calculated using the same basic formula used to calculate static friction: $fk=\mu kFn$ with the only differences being the sub-k marks replacing the sub-s marks of the previous equation, signifying kinetic friction.

As kinetic friction slows an object, the object's kinetic energy is transformed into heat.

Fundamental Forces: Electromagnetism

Electromagnetism is one of the four fundamental forces. It is far more common than gravity, but only if you know where to look.

Electromagnetism is responsible for nearly all interactions in which gravity plays no part. It is what holds negatively charged electrons in orbit around the positively charged protons in the nucleus of an atom. It is also the force that joins atoms to each other to create molecules.

It is also electromagnetism that is responsible for the fact that matter—which is made up of atoms and at the subatomic level is mostly empty space—feels solid.

When you sit down in your chair, it is the electromagnetic attraction between the chair's atoms and between your body's atoms that keep you from falling through the chair and, conversely, that keep the chair from passing through you.

Electromagnetic force acts through a field.

This type of field can occur as a result of positively or negatively charged atoms (ions), atoms which have either more or fewer electrons than protons causing their overall charge to be unbalanced. Magnetic fields can also be created by applying electric current to conductive material (such as wire) with a conductive core (such as a nail).

Electric current is nothing more than a steady flow of electrons, and by turning on the current you send electrons through the core.

This aligns all the atoms in the metal so that they are parallel with each other, and this creates a magnetic field. When you turn the electric current off, the electrons stop flowing, and the atoms, no longer forced by the current to line up, cease to be magnetic.

All electromagnetic fields have a positive and a negative pole.

Even the Earth's magnetic field, which is caused by the convective forces in the planet's core, sends electrons out of its negative pole (in the geographic North Pole) and reaccepts them at its positive pole (in the geographic South Pole in Antarctica). The Earth's magnetic field, like all magnetic fields, is able to affect charged particles.

Magnetic fields move in one direction around a magnet.

This direction is always the same in relation to the flow of current from the negative to the positive poles, and it is easy to test the direction of the field using the "right hand rule." Close your fist and make a "thumbs up" sign with your right hand. The positive pole is represented by the tip of your thumb, the negative by the other end of your hand, and the direction of the magnetic field by where your closed fingers are. Thus, if you point your thumb at yourself, your magnet has current coming out its negative pole pointed towards you and looping back around to the positive pole pointed away from you, and the field is pointed counter-clockwise, which, here, is to your left.

The effects of a magnetic field do not go on forever but follow the inverse square law.

The farther you move from a magnetic field, the less its force will affect you. By moving x times away from a magnetic field, you feel 1/x2 times less magnetism.

Closely related to the electromagnetic field is electromagnetic radiation.

This radiation can take many forms, the most familiar of which being light, radio waves that carry radio and broadcast television, microwaves that cook our food, x-rays that can image the insides or our bodies, and gamma rays that come down from space and would have killed us all long ago if it were not for the Earth's magnetic field interacting with them.

Electromagnetic radiation is created, according to James Clerk Maxwell, by the oscillations of electromagnetic fields, which create electromagnetic waves.

The wave's frequency (or how energetic it is) determines what part of the electromagnetic spectrum it occupies—whether it is a gamma ray, a blue light or a radio signal. Electromagnetic radiation is the same thing as light, with what we are used to as visible light being a range of specific frequencies within the electromagnetic spectrum, so all electromagnetic radiation moves at the speed of light.

At the quantum level, the electromagnetic force has a transfer particle moving back and forth between charged atoms, attracting and repelling them. The electromagnetic transfer particle is the photon.

Fundamental Forces: Gravity

Gravity may be the most commonly, consciously experienced force.

We can see its effects everyday when books fall off shelves, when stray baseballs arc downwards and crash through windows and when Australians time and again fail to fall off the bottom of the world and out into space. Gravity is also largely responsible for the structure of the universe. Without it, stars would not ignite and begin fusion reactions, planets would not condense out of dust and metal and most matter would have no attraction to other matter in any way. Without gravity, life would not exist.

It may seem strange to learn that gravity is the weakest of all forces given that it holds the entire galaxy together.

Still, even with the gravitational mass of the entire planet pulling on an object such as a ball—causing it to sit motionless on the floor rather than float aimlessly off into space—a toddler could easily pick it up and run off with it, and there would be nothing the planet could do about it. Match that with the force an electromagnet exerts on metal; there is no comparison.

The idea of gravity as a force was first formulated by Isaac Newton in the late 17th century.

Newton's ideas were further elaborated on in the early 20th century by Albert Einstein, who described gravity as the effect of mass warping the fabric of space-time. This process is often portrayed as a large ball creating a divot in a flat sheet of space-time. The divot curves space-time and can catch objects that would otherwise be traveling in straight lines and redirect or even capture them.

On Earth gravity pulls objects towards the center of the planet at $9.8 m/s^2$.

The squared rate of time shows that gravity is by its nature a force causing acceleration. Every second, the force of gravity increases the speed of an object by an additional 9.8m/s, provided nothing able to resist the force gets in its way.

In Einstein's view of the universe, gravity moved in waves, which traveled through space at the speed of light.

As a result, he demonstrated that the force of gravity would take time to reach the object it was acting on. If, for instance, the sun were to vanish suddenly from the solar system, it would take eight minutes for the Earth to go flying off into space—the same amount of time it would take for us to stop seeing the sun's light.

Another way to view gravity is through a series of transfer particles that interact with matter and draw it closer together.

Transfer particles come into play in quantum mechanics, and they replace gravity waves as the method of spreading the force through the universe. (Actually, replace is not the right word, as quantum mechanics shows that particles and waves are really the same thing, simply looked at from different perspectives.) In quantum mechanics gravity's transfer particle is called a graviton, and it moves at the speed of light.

The farther you move from a gravitational mass, the less its force will affect you.

The drop in the gravitational force is governed by what is known as the inverse square law, which says that the attraction of any object drops in relation to the square of the distance you move from it. If you are floating over the surface of the planet and then move x times away from it, you will feel $1/x^2$ times less gravity. So if you move 10 times farther away from where you were, you will feel 1/100 the force gravity.

Fundamental Forces: Strong and Weak Nuclear Forces

The strong and weak nuclear forces are fundamental forces, but they were discovered much later than electromagnetism and gravity primarily because they only interact with matter at a subatomic level.

Strong nuclear force is the strongest of the four fundamental forces.

Strong nuclear force is 100 times stronger than the next strongest force, electromagnetism, and 1036 times the strength of the weakest force, gravity. That said, for the thousands of years that people have been studying physics, it never occurred to anyone to even look for the strong force. That is because, despite the strong force's strength, it has such a limited range that it only interacts with matter across the distance of an atom's nucleus. In fact, its range is only about 10-15 meters, so small that the nuclei of the largest atoms—those filled with the highest number of protons and neutrons—are only just barely small enough for the strong force to keep working, making the nuclei of those atoms unstable.

The strong force was not discovered until the 1930s when scientists discovered the neutron.

Until that time atomic nuclei were thought to consist of a collection of protons and electrons grouped together in such a way that kept them mutually attracted. With the discovery of the neutron, however, a new force was needed to hold positively charged protons together with uncharged neutrons.

Strong Nuclear force interacts with Quarks.

The strong force actually does not interact directly with the protons and neutrons but with the fundamental particle that makes up protons and neutrons, quarks. Quarks come in three different color groupings: red, green and blue. (Quarks are not actually these colors; red, green and blue are just familiar names given to bits of matter that are utterly outside our experience as humans, to make them easier to comprehend.) The different colors of quarks combine to create protons and neutrons. Within each proton and neutron, the strong force holds the quarks together. That, in turn, bleeds out into the rest of the nucleus in a residual effect, holding the protons and neutrons together as well.

Like the other fundamental forces, the strong force is mediated at the quantum level using a transfer particle known as a gluon. However, unlike the transfer particles for gravity and electromagnetism (gravitons and photons, respectively), gluons have mass. It is the gluon's mass that limits the area where it can spread the strong force to only within the nucleus.

Weak nuclear force causes a type of radioactive decay.

The other fundamental force operating inside the nucleus is the weak force. The weak force causes a specific type of radioactive decay called beta decay, so named because it causes the decaying atom to emit a beta particle, which can be either an electron or a positron (a form of anti-mater also known as an anti-electron), as a byproduct of changing into a different element.

Several things happen at once during beta decay, and we should look at each one individually. We saw while looking at the strong force that an atom's protons and neutrons are made up of smaller, fundamental particles called quarks, and it is the quarks that actually interact with the strong force. As it turns out, quarks are the only particle that interacts with all four fundamental forces, which means that inside the nucleus they are interacting with the weak force as well.

In addition to three different colors: red, blue and green, Quarks can be divided into six different flavors: up, down, charm, strange, top and bottom.

Before we get to how the weak force interacts with quarks, there is something else you should understand. We mentioned above that quarks come in three different colors: red, blue and green. However, they also can be divided into six different flavors: up, down, charm, strange, top and bottom. (This makes 18 different possible combinations of quark, each with a color and a flavor.) Of these flavors only up and down quarks are stable enough to form protons and neutrons.

What the weak force does is switch up quarks to down quarks and down quarks to up quarks.

This is the only thing that the weak force does, but it has several effects. First since quarks join to produce protons and neutrons (two up quarks and one down quark make a proton, while two down and one up quark make a neutron), the sudden change of one type of quark to another, changes that combination. $\beta-$ decay is beta decay where change of quarks causes a neutron to become a proton. This also causes the atom to emit an electron and a electron antineutrino. $\beta +$ decay is the opposite, where a proton changes to a neutron and the atom emits a positron and an electron neutrino.

In both cases the decaying atom changes into a different kind of atom. In general, beta decay takes place in unstable isotopes (atoms that have a different number of protons and neutrons) and stabilizes the nucleus by equalizing the ratio of these particles. For instance, beta decay will turn the unstable plutonium 15 into far more stable strontium 16.

Quantum Mechanics

Quantum mechanics is the study of quanta, the most basic individual unit of any substance.

Quantum mechanics began as a discipline within physics in 1900 when Max Planck determined that energy radiated as heat could not just radiate at any old temperature it wanted, but that it could only rise and fall—and thus be emitted or absorbed—at certain, set levels. (Think of it as the difference between stairs and ramps. Stairs have set spaces where you can stand and set spaces where you cannot. Planck said that raising energy levels such as temperature was akin to climbing a set of stairs one step at a time.)

Radiation that produces heat (and thus all electromagnetic radiation, including visible light) is made up of tiny little particles, which Planck named quanta from the Latin work "quantus," which means "how much."

Planck developed an equation to describe this situation, $E=hv$ in which v stood for the already well known frequencies of electromagnetic spectrum (and which in 1900 was thought of as only acting like a wave), h stood for a number called the Planck constant that equaled $6.63\times10-34$ J s ("J s" is for Joule seconds), and E was the energy level for quanta of that frequency.

In 1905 Albert Einstein used Planck's work to define the photon, which is one quantum of electromagnetic radiation.

Photons are generally thought of as light, but only some energies of photons are visible. Photons can have any energy that corresponds to electromagnetic frequency, but instead of being a continuous wave, they are thought of as individual particles.

Waves and particles are the same thing look at in different ways.

The discovery of the particle aspect of a wave led to a realization that waves and particles were actually the same thing, looked at in different ways. This idea, called wave-particle duality, accounted for the centuries long debate between physicists over whether light was a wave or a particle, with each side producing compelling evidence to prove its thesis. As it turned out light—like everything in the universe—was both. This relationship was demonstrated by Louis de Broglie who developed the equation $p=h/\lambda$ showing that the Planck constant (h) divided by a particle's wavelength (λ, pronounced lambda) would equal its momentum (p). Since all particles are moving and have momentum, all particles have wavelengths.

One of the most important aspects of wave-particle duality comes from studying atoms.

The orbits of electrons around the atomic nuclei had at one time been thought to mimic the orbits of planets around the sun. Now, however, two important factors came into play to change that view. The first was the realization that electrons could only orbit at certain distances from the nucleus. When changing from one electron shell to the next, an electron would not take a gradual trajectory to its new home in the way a spaceship from Earth to Mars might. The electron would simply vanish from one shell and appear instantaneously at the next. In essence, electrons could also only display certain quanta of energy. They could have one energy level or another, but they could not exist in between.

The second important thing that quantum mechanics showed physicists is that "orbit" does not describe electrons and is only symbolic.

Since all particles are also waves, an electron could not simply be in one place at one time, but had to exist as across a range of areas as a frequency which described its momentum.

The Heisenberg uncertainty principle states you can measure the position of an electron or the velocity, but not both at once.

This seemingly nonsensical idea was explained mathematically though the Heisenberg uncertainty principle, which stated that it was possible to measure the exact position of a particle, and it was possible to measure the exact velocity of a particle, but you could not know both factors at once. In other words, measuring one would make it impossible to measure the other. This was an unavoidable fact of reality given de Broglie's equation; if you were moving you were spread out like a wave.

No particles in the universe can be said to have definite positions in space.

A strange side effect of this was it meant that no particles in the universe could be said to have definite positions in space. Instead, everything had a likely position given its velocity. Matter could not be said to exist at certain points in space, it could merely have certain probabilities of existing at those points.

Gravity is still a problem.

The 21st century understanding of gravity comes from Einstein's work on Special and General Relativity. The various predictions made by Einstein's theories have been proven correct experimentally on numerous occasions, and clearly his ideas accurately explain reality. However, they do not mix with quantum mechanics.

Physics has three zones which do not mix - relativity, quantum mechanics and Newtonian.

It is possible to look at physics and think of there as being three distinct zones: relativity, which describes the very big and the very fast; quantum mechanics, which describes the very small; and Newtonian physics, which describes everything in between.

But Newtonian physics easily unifies with quantum theory since the chaos and weirdness at the individual wave-particle level smooths out as you add more and more particles together, which is what we see when we look at the macro world in which we live. (That is, when you look at an object in front of you, you see it existing in a definite point in space because many particles make it up the probability that they will all end suddenly existing elsewhere—the way individual particles can—drops to nearly zero.) Additionally, three of the four fundamental forces, electromagnetism, the strong force and the weak force, can all be explained through quantum mechanics using their three transfer particles; photons, gluons and bosons. They have been unified. However, the use of a gravity transfer particle, the graviton, in models has been less successful at bringing the experimentally accurate predictions of relativity in line with the functioning of reality at the quantum level.

States of Matter

Matter on Earth can exist in three main states or phases: solid, liquid and gas. There is also a fourth phase, plasma, that occurs when matter is superheated.

The primary difference between the different phases of matter is the behavior of molecules relative to the temperature the matter is exposed to. The lower the temperature, the closer together and more locked together the molecules are. The higher the temperature, the farther apart the molecules are and the more they move relative to each other.

Solid

Solid matter exists in a state where its molecules are locked together in a rigid structure preventing them from moving and, as a result, solid matter is held together in a specific shape.

There are two primary types of solids, each defined by the structures in which their molecules are held. When the molecules in solid matter maintain a uniform organization they form a polycrystalline structure. This is how molecules in metal, ice and salt are organized. Polycrystalline structures are generally a result of the molecules' ionic properties. Water molecules, for instance, are formed in such a way that there are distinct ends, one with two hydrogen atoms and one with a single oxygen atom. The structure of the atoms within a water molecule means these ends are charged, giving it what amount to poles and causing water molecules to join only in specific patterns. Under a microscope polycrystalline solids are generally described as resembling lattice work or a chain link fence, with the same pattern of molecules from one end to the other.

When molecule's electromagnetic properties do not incline them to form into particular structures, they glob together in whatever patterns they can. This produces amorphous solids, most notably foams, glass and many types of plastic. Amorphous solids have no regular pattern throughout their structure and, as a result, are poor conductors of heat and electricity.

Liquid

When solids are heated past a certain point, the electromagnetic bonds holding their molecules together loosen, and the molecules are able to move more freely.

While the temperatures required for this to happen can vary widely, the particular physical qualities of a liquid are always the same. Liquids are considered to be fluids, which differ from solids primarily in their ability to take the shape of any container they are held in. This is the result of a less intense electromagnetic connection between the molecules than there is in solids; however, there is still enough that liquids still want to stay all in the same place. This is why liquids still maintain a low density that is nearly identical to their densities in solid form, and why they will maintain a constant volume rather than just drift off the way gasses do.

Liquids also have a property known as viscosity, which describes their willingness to flow over and away from themselves. Liquids such as water and honey have a constant viscosity and are known as Newtonian fluids. Non-Newtonian fluids, such as a goopy mixture of water and cornstarch can change their viscosities.

Gas

The third state of matter that is commonly found on Earth is gas. Gasses are formed when matter is heated beyond its liquid state so that the electromagnetic bonds holding its molecules together are severed almost completely.

Gasses are also considered fluids and like liquids have no definite shape. However, unlike liquids they also lack a definite volume and have an extremely low density compared to their solid forms.

Since gasses lack both a shape and a volume, they will expand to fill any container they are placed in. Left unbounded they will expand forever. Conversely, gasses are perfectly happy to compress together in an enclosed space. (However, the more molecules of a gas that are enclosed in a space together, the higher the gas's pressure—the force exerted by the molecules on the container's surface—will be.) One interesting thing about this expansion and compression is that it will always be homogeneous, meaning that as a gas expands to fill a container, there will never be pockets of a higher density of molecules in some areas with a lower density of molecules in others. The molecules will expand to fill the container equally.

Plasma

Plasma is the next step up from a gas; it is when a gas' molecules become super heated to the point where the molecular bonds themselves break down and the atoms begin shedding their electrons.

Although plasma is rarely found on Earth, it is the most common state of matter throughout the universe. (It is the primary state of matter in stars, for instance.) Plasma has some unique characteristics, not the least of which is that it is ionized, or electrically charged. In many ways plasma acts like a gas. It lacks any definite shape or volume, and it will homogenously fill any container. However, it can also be manipulated by electromagnetic fields, which alters its shape or contain it. Plasma is a super-heated, magnetically charged gas.

Practice Test Questions Set 1

THE PRACTICE TEST PORTION PRESENTS QUESTIONS THAT ARE REPRESENTATIVE OF THE TYPE OF QUESTION YOU SHOULD EXPECT TO FIND ON THE DET. However, they are not intended to match exactly what is on the DET.

For the best results, take this Practice Test as if it were the real exam. Set aside time when you will not be disturbed, and a location that is quiet and free of distractions. Read the instructions carefully, read each question carefully, and answer to the best of your ability.

Use the bubble answer sheets provided. When you have completed the Practice Test, check your answer against the Answer Key and read the explanation provided.

NOTE: The Science, Anatomy and Physiology and English sections are optional. Check with your school for exam details.

Reading Comprehension Answer Sheet

1. Ⓐ Ⓑ Ⓒ Ⓓ	18. Ⓐ Ⓑ Ⓒ Ⓓ	35. Ⓐ Ⓑ Ⓒ Ⓓ
2. Ⓐ Ⓑ Ⓒ Ⓓ	19. Ⓐ Ⓑ Ⓒ Ⓓ	36. Ⓐ Ⓑ Ⓒ Ⓓ
3. Ⓐ Ⓑ Ⓒ Ⓓ	20. Ⓐ Ⓑ Ⓒ Ⓓ	37. Ⓐ Ⓑ Ⓒ Ⓓ
4. Ⓐ Ⓑ Ⓒ Ⓓ	21. Ⓐ Ⓑ Ⓒ Ⓓ	38. Ⓐ Ⓑ Ⓒ Ⓓ
5. Ⓐ Ⓑ Ⓒ Ⓓ	22. Ⓐ Ⓑ Ⓒ Ⓓ	39. Ⓐ Ⓑ Ⓒ Ⓓ
6. Ⓐ Ⓑ Ⓒ Ⓓ	23. Ⓐ Ⓑ Ⓒ Ⓓ	40. Ⓐ Ⓑ Ⓒ Ⓓ
7. Ⓐ Ⓑ Ⓒ Ⓓ	24. Ⓐ Ⓑ Ⓒ Ⓓ	
8. Ⓐ Ⓑ Ⓒ Ⓓ	25. Ⓐ Ⓑ Ⓒ Ⓓ	
9. Ⓐ Ⓑ Ⓒ Ⓓ	26. Ⓐ Ⓑ Ⓒ Ⓓ	
10. Ⓐ Ⓑ Ⓒ Ⓓ	27. Ⓐ Ⓑ Ⓒ Ⓓ	
11. Ⓐ Ⓑ Ⓒ Ⓓ	28. Ⓐ Ⓑ Ⓒ Ⓓ	
12. Ⓐ Ⓑ Ⓒ Ⓓ	29. Ⓐ Ⓑ Ⓒ Ⓓ	
13. Ⓐ Ⓑ Ⓒ Ⓓ	30. Ⓐ Ⓑ Ⓒ Ⓓ	
14. Ⓐ Ⓑ Ⓒ Ⓓ	31. Ⓐ Ⓑ Ⓒ Ⓓ	
15. Ⓐ Ⓑ Ⓒ Ⓓ	32. Ⓐ Ⓑ Ⓒ Ⓓ	
16. Ⓐ Ⓑ Ⓒ Ⓓ	33. Ⓐ Ⓑ Ⓒ Ⓓ	
17. Ⓐ Ⓑ Ⓒ Ⓓ	34. Ⓐ Ⓑ Ⓒ Ⓓ	

Math Answer Sheet

1. A B C D
2. A B C D
3. A B C D
4. A B C D
5. A B C D
6. A B C D
7. A B C D
8. A B C D
9. A B C D
10. A B C D
11. A B C D
12. A B C D
13. A B C D
14. A B C D
15. A B C D
16. A B C D
17. A B C D
18. A B C D
19. A B C D
20. A B C D
21. A B C D
22. A B C D
23. A B C D
24. A B C D
25. A B C D
26. A B C D
27. A B C D
28. A B C D
29. A B C D
30. A B C D
31. A B C D
32. A B C D
33. A B C D
34. A B C D
35. A B C D
36. A B C D
37. A B C D
38. A B C D
39. A B C D
40. A B C D
41. A B C D
42. A B C D
43. A B C D
44. A B C D
45. A B C D
46. A B C D
47. A B C D
48. A B C D
49. A B C D
50. A B C D

English Answer Sheet

1. (A) (B) (C) (D)
2. (A) (B) (C) (D)
3. (A) (B) (C) (D)
4. (A) (B) (C) (D)
5. (A) (B) (C) (D)
6. (A) (B) (C) (D)
7. (A) (B) (C) (D)
8. (A) (B) (C) (D)
9. (A) (B) (C) (D)
10. (A) (B) (C) (D)
11. (A) (B) (C) (D)
12. (A) (B) (C) (D)
13. (A) (B) (C) (D)
14. (A) (B) (C) (D)
15. (A) (B) (C) (D)
16. (A) (B) (C) (D)
17. (A) (B) (C) (D)
18. (A) (B) (C) (D)
19. (A) (B) (C) (D)
20. (A) (B) (C) (D)
21. (A) (B) (C) (D)
22. (A) (B) (C) (D)
23. (A) (B) (C) (D)
24. (A) (B) (C) (D)
25. (A) (B) (C) (D)
26. (A) (B) (C) (D)
27. (A) (B) (C) (D)
28. (A) (B) (C) (D)
29. (A) (B) (C) (D)
30. (A) (B) (C) (D)
31. (A) (B) (C) (D)
32. (A) (B) (C) (D)
33. (A) (B) (C) (D)
34. (A) (B) (C) (D)
35. (A) (B) (C) (D)
36. (A) (B) (C) (D)
37. (A) (B) (C) (D)
38. (A) (B) (C) (D)
39. (A) (B) (C) (D)
40. (A) (B) (C) (D)
41. (A) (B) (C) (D)
42. (A) (B) (C) (D)
43. (A) (B) (C) (D)
44. (A) (B) (C) (D)
45. (A) (B) (C) (D)
46. (A) (B) (C) (D)
47. (A) (B) (C) (D)
48. (A) (B) (C) (D)
49. (A) (B) (C) (D)
50. (A) (B) (C) (D)

Critical Thinking Answer Sheet

1. (A) (B) (C) (D)
2. (A) (B) (C) (D)
3. (A) (B) (C) (D)
4. (A) (B) (C) (D)
5. (A) (B) (C) (D)
6. (A) (B) (C) (D)
7. (A) (B) (C) (D)
8. (A) (B) (C) (D)
9. (A) (B) (C) (D)
10. (A) (B) (C) (D)
11. (A) (B) (C) (D)
12. (A) (B) (C) (D)
13. (A) (B) (C) (D)
14. (A) (B) (C) (D)
15. (A) (B) (C) (D)
16. (A) (B) (C) (D)
17. (A) (B) (C) (D)
18. (A) (B) (C) (D)
19. (A) (B) (C) (D)
20. (A) (B) (C) (D)

Science Answer Sheet

1. (A) (B) (C) (D)
2. (A) (B) (C) (D)
3. (A) (B) (C) (D)
4. (A) (B) (C) (D)
5. (A) (B) (C) (D)
6. (A) (B) (C) (D)
7. (A) (B) (C) (D)
8. (A) (B) (C) (D)
9. (A) (B) (C) (D)
10. (A) (B) (C) (D)
11. (A) (B) (C) (D)
12. (A) (B) (C) (D)
13. (A) (B) (C) (D)
14. (A) (B) (C) (D)
15. (A) (B) (C) (D)
16. (A) (B) (C) (D)
17. (A) (B) (C) (D)
18. (A) (B) (C) (D)
19. (A) (B) (C) (D)
20. (A) (B) (C) (D)
21. (A) (B) (C) (D)
22. (A) (B) (C) (D)
23. (A) (B) (C) (D)
24. (A) (B) (C) (D)
25. (A) (B) (C) (D)
26. (A) (B) (C) (D)
27. (A) (B) (C) (D)
28. (A) (B) (C) (D)
29. (A) (B) (C) (D)
30. (A) (B) (C) (D)
31. (A) (B) (C) (D)
32. (A) (B) (C) (D)
33. (A) (B) (C) (D)
34. (A) (B) (C) (D)
35. (A) (B) (C) (D)
36. (A) (B) (C) (D)
37. (A) (B) (C) (D)
38. (A) (B) (C) (D)
39. (A) (B) (C) (D)
40. (A) (B) (C) (D)
41. (A) (B) (C) (D)
42. (A) (B) (C) (D)
43. (A) (B) (C) (D)
44. (A) (B) (C) (D)
45. (A) (B) (C) (D)
46. (A) (B) (C) (D)
47. (A) (B) (C) (D)
48. (A) (B) (C) (D)
49. (A) (B) (C) (D)
50. (A) (B) (C) (D)

Section I - Reading Comprehension.

Directions: The following questions are based on several reading passages. Each passage is followed by a series of questions. Read each passage carefully, and then answer the questions based on it. You may reread the passage as often as you wish. When you have finished answering the questions based on one passage, go right on to the next passage. Choose the best answer based on the information given and implied.

Questions 1 – 4 refer to the following passage.

Passage 1 - Infectious Disease

An infectious disease is a clinically evident illness resulting from the presence of pathogenic agents, such as viruses, bacteria, fungi, protozoa, multicellular parasites, and unusual proteins known as prions. Infectious pathologies are also called communicable diseases or transmissible diseases, due to their potential of transmission from one person or species to another by a replicating agent (as opposed to a toxin).

Transmission of an infectious disease can occur in many different ways. Physical contact, liquids, food, body fluids, contaminated objects, and airborne inhalation can all transmit infecting agents.

Transmissible diseases that occur through contact with an ill person, or objects touched by them, are especially infective, and are sometimes called contagious diseases. Communicable diseases that require a more specialized route of infection, such as through blood or needle transmission, or sexual transmission, are usually not regarded as contagious.

The term infectivity describes the ability of an organism to enter, survive and multiply in the host, while the infectiousness of a disease shows the comparative ease with which the disease is transmitted. An infection however, is not synonymous with an infectious disease, as an infection may not cause important clinical symptoms. [10]

1. What can we infer from the first paragraph in this passage?

a. Sickness from a toxin can be easily transmitted from one person to another.

b. Sickness from an infectious disease can be easily transmitted from one person to another.

c. Few sicknesses are transmitted from one person to another.

d. Infectious diseases are easily treated.

2. What are two other names for infections' pathologies?

a. Communicable diseases or transmissible diseases

b. Communicable diseases or terminal diseases

c. Transmissible diseases or preventable diseases

d. Communicative diseases or unstable diseases

3. What does infectivity describe?

a. The inability of an organism to multiply in the host.
b. The inability of an organism to reproduce.
c. The ability of an organism to enter, survive and multiply in the host.
d. The ability of an organism to reproduce in the host.

4. How do we know an infection is not synonymous with an infectious disease?

a. Because an infectious disease destroys infections with enough time.
b. Because an infection may not cause important clinical symptoms or impair host function.
c. We do not. The two are synonymous.
d. Because an infection is too fatal to be an infectious disease.

Questions 5 – 8 refer to the following passage.

Low Blood Sugar

As the name suggest, low blood sugar is low sugar levels in the bloodstream. This can occur when you have not eaten properly and undertake strenuous activity, or, when you are very hungry. When Low blood sugar occurs regularly and is ongoing, it is a medical condition called hypoglycemia. This condition can occur in diabetics and in healthy adults.

Causes of low blood sugar can include excessive alcohol consumption, metabolic problems, stomach surgery, pancreas, liver or kidneys problems, as well as a side-effect of some medications.

Symptoms

There are different symptoms depending on the severity of the case.

Mild hypoglycemia can lead to feelings of nausea and hunger. The patient may also feel nervous, jittery and have fast heart beats. Sweaty skin, clammy and cold skin are likely symptoms.

Moderate hypoglycemia can result in short temperedness, confusion, nervousness, fear and blurring of vision. The patient may feel weak and unsteady.

Severe cases of hypoglycemia can lead to seizures, coma, fainting spells, nightmares, headaches, excessive sweats and severe tiredness.

Diagnosis of low blood sugar

A doctor can diagnosis this medical condition by asking the patient questions and testing blood and urine samples. Home testing kits are available for patients to monitor blood sugar levels. It is important to see a qualified doctor though. The doctor can administer tests to ensure that will safely rule out other medical conditions that could affect blood sugar levels.

Treatment

Quick treatments include drinking or eating foods and drinks with high sugar contents. Good examples include soda, fruit juice, hard candy and raisins. Glucose energy tablets can also help. Doctors may also recommend medications and well as changes in diet and exercise routine to treat chronic low blood sugar.

5. Based on the article, which of the following is true?

a. Low blood sugar can happen to anyone.
b. Low blood sugar only happens to diabetics.
c. Low blood sugar can occur even.
d. None of the statements are true.

6. Which of the following are the author's opinion?

a. Quick treatments include drinking or eating foods and drinks with high sugar contents.
b. None of the statements are opinions.
c. This condition can occur in diabetics and in healthy adults.
d. There are different symptoms depending on the severity of the case

7. What is the author's purpose?

a. To inform
b. To persuade
c. To entertain
d. To analyze

8. Which of the following is not a detail?

a. A doctor can diagnosis this medical condition by asking the patient questions and testing.
b. A doctor will test blood and urine samples.
c. Glucose energy tablets can also help.
d. Home test kits monitor blood sugar levels.

Questions 9 – 11 refer to the following passage.

Passage 3 – Thunderstorms

The first stage of a thunderstorm is the cumulus stage, or developing stage. In this stage, masses of moisture are lifted upwards into the atmosphere. The trigger for this lift can be insulation heating the ground producing thermals, areas where two winds converge, forcing air upwards, or, where winds blow over terrain of increasing elevation. Moisture in the air rapidly cools into liquid drops of water, which appears as cumulus clouds.

As the water vapor condenses into liquid, latent heat is released which warms the air, causing it to become less dense than the surrounding dry air. The warm air rises in an updraft through the process of convection (hence the term convective precipitation). This creates a low-pressure zone beneath the forming thunderstorm. In a typical thunderstorm, about 5×10^8 kg of water vapor is lifted, and the quantity of energy released when this condenses is about equal to the energy used by a city of 100,000 in a month. [11]

9. The cumulus stage of a thunderstorm is the

a. The last stage of the storm.
b. The middle stage of the storm formation.
c. The beginning of the thunderstorm.
d. The period after the thunderstorm has ended.

10. One of the ways the air is warmed is

a. Air moving downwards, which creates a high-pressure zone.
b. Air cooling and becoming less dense, causing it to rise.
c. Moisture moving downward toward the earth.
d. Heat created by water vapor condensing into liquid.

11. Identify the correct sequence of events

a. Warm air rises, water droplets condense, creating more heat, and the air rises farther.

b. Warm air rises and cools, water droplets condense, causing low pressure.

c. Warm air rises and collects water vapor, the water vapor condenses as the air rises, which creates heat, and causes the air to rise farther.

d. None of the above.

Questions 12 – 14 refer to the following passage.

Passage 4 If You Have Allergies, You're Not Alone

People who experience allergies might joke that their immune systems have let them down or are seriously lacking. Truthfully though, people who experience allergic reactions or allergy symptoms during certain times of the year have heightened immune systems that are "better" than those of people who have perfectly healthy but less militant immune systems.

Still, when a person has an allergic reaction, they are having an adverse reaction to a substance that is considered normal to most people. Mild allergic reactions usually have symptoms like itching, runny nose, red eyes, or bumps or discoloration of the skin. More serious allergic reactions, such as those to animal and insect poisons or certain foods, may result in the closing of the throat, swelling of the eyes, low blood pressure, an inability to breath, and can even be fatal.

Different treatments help different allergies, and which one a person uses depends on the nature and severity of the allergy. It is recommended to patients with severe allergies to take extra precautions, such as carrying an EpiPen, which treats anaphylactic shock and may prevent death, always in order for the remedy to be readily available and more effective. When an allergy is not so severe, treatments may be used just relieve a person of uncomfortable symptoms. Over the counter allergy medicines treat milder symptoms, and can be bought at any grocery store and used in moderation to help people with allergies live normally.

There are many tests available to assess whether a person has allergies or what they may be allergic to, and advances in these tests and the medicine used to treat patients continues to improve. Despite this fact, allergies still affect many people throughout the year or even every day. Medicines used to treat allergies have side effects of their own, and it is difficult to bring the body into balance with the use of medicine. Regardless, many of those who live with allergies are grateful for what is available and find it useful in maintaining their lifestyles.

12. According to this passage, it can be understood that the word "militant" belongs in a group with the words:

a. sickly, ailing, faint

b. strength, power, vigor

c. active, fighting, warring

d. worn, tired, breaking down

13. The author says that "medicines used to treat allergies have side effects of their own" to

a. point out that doctors aren't very good at diagnosing and treating allergies

b. argue that because of the large number of people with allergies, a cure will never be found

c. explain that allergy medicines aren't cures and some compromise must be made

d. argue that more wholesome remedies should be researched and medicines banned

14. It can be inferred that ______ recommend that some people with allergies carry medicine with them.

a. the author

b. doctors

c. the makers of EpiPen

d. people with allergies

Questions 15 refers to the following Table of Contents.

Contents

15. Consider the table of contents above. What page would you find information about natural selection and adaptation?

a. 81

b. 90

c. 110

d. 132

Questions 16 – 19 refer to the following passage.

Passage 5 - Clouds

A cloud is a visible mass of droplets or frozen crystals floating in the atmosphere above the surface of the Earth or other planetary bodies. Another type of cloud is a mass of material in space, attracted by gravity, called interstellar clouds and nebulae. The branch of meteorology which studies clouds is called nephrology. When we are speaking of Earth clouds, water vapor is usually the condensing substance, which forms small droplets or ice crystal. These crystals are typically 0.01 mm in diameter. Dense, deep clouds reflect most light, so they appear white, at least from the top. Cloud droplets scatter light very efficiently, so the farther into a cloud light travels, the weaker it gets. This accounts for the gray or dark appearance at the base of large clouds. Thin clouds may appear to have acquired the color of their environment or background. [12]

16. What are clouds made of?

a. Water droplets
b. Ice crystals
c. Ice crystals and water droplets
d. Clouds on Earth are made of ice crystals and water droplets

17. The main idea of this passage is

a. Condensation occurs in clouds, having an intense effect on the weather on the surface of the earth.

b. Atmospheric gases are responsible for the gray color of clouds just before a severe storm happens.

c. A cloud is a visible mass of droplets or frozen crystals floating in the atmosphere above the surface of the Earth or other planetary body.

d. Clouds reflect light in varying amounts and degrees, depending on the size and concentration of the water droplets.

18. The branch of meteorology that studies clouds is called

a. Convection
b. Thermal meteorology
c. Nephology
d. Nephelometry

19. Why are clouds white on top and grey on the bottom?

a. Because water droplets inside the cloud do not reflect light, it appears white, and the farther into the cloud the light travels, the less light is reflected making the bottom appear dark.

b. Because water droplets outside the cloud reflect light, it appears dark, and the farther into the cloud the light travels, the more light is reflected making the bottom appear white.

c. Because water droplets inside the cloud reflects light, making it appear white, and the farther into the cloud the light travels, the more light is reflected making the bottom appear dark.

d. None of the above.

Questions 20 - 23 refer to the following recipe.

"When a Poet Longs to Mourn, He Writes an Elegy"

Poems are an expressive, especially emotional, form of writing. They have been present in literature virtually from the time civilizations invented the written word. Poets often portrayed as moody, secluded, and even troubled, but this is because poets are introspective and feel deeply about the current events and cultural norms they are surrounded with. Poets often produce the most telling literature, giving insight into the society and mindset they come from. This can be done in many forms.

The oldest types of poems often include many stanzas, may or may not rhyme, and are more about telling a story than experimenting with language or words. The most common types of ancient poetry are epics, which are usually extremely long stories that follow a hero through his journey, or ellegies, which are often solemn in tone and used to mourn or lament something or someone. The Mesopotamians are often said to have invented the written word, and their literature is among the oldest in the world, including the epic poem titled "Epic of Gilgamesh." Similar in style and length to "Gilgamesh" is "Beowulf," an ellegy poem written in Old English and set in Scandinavia. These poems are often used by professors as the earliest examples of literature.

The importance of poetry was revived in the Renaissance. At this time, Europeans discovered the style and beauty of ancient Greek arts, and poetry was among those. Shakespeare is the most well-known poet of the time, and he used poetry not only to write poems but also to write plays for the theater. The most popular forms of poetry during the Renaissance included villanelles, sonnets, as well as the epic. Poets during this time focused on style and form, and developed very specific rules and outlines for how an exceptional poem should be written.

As often happens in the arts, modern poets have rejected the constricting rules of Renaissance poets, and free form poems are much more popular. Some modern poems would read just like stories if they weren't arranged into lines and stanzas. It is difficult to tell which poems and poets will be the most important, because works of art often become more famous in hindsight, after the poet has died and society can look at itself without being in the moment. Modern poetry continues to develop, and will no doubt continue to change as values, thought, and writing continue to change.

Poems can be among the most enlightening and uplifting texts for a person to read if they are looking to connect with the past, connect with other people, or try to gain an understanding of what is happening in their time.

20. In summary, the author has written this passage

a. as a foreword that will introduce a poem in a book or magazine

b. because she loves poetry and wants more people to like it

c. to give a brief history of poems

d. in order to convince students to write poems

21. The author organizes the paragraphs mainly by

a. moving chronologically, explaining which types of poetry were common in that time

b. talking about new types of poems each paragraph and explaining them a little

c. focusing on one poet or group of people and the poems they wrote

d. explaining older types of poetry so she can talk about modern poetry

22. The author's claim that poetry has been around "virtually from the time civilizations invented the written word" is supported by the detail that

a. Beowulf is written in Old English, which is not really in use any longer

b. epic poems told stories about heroes

c. the Renaissance poets tried to copy Greek poets

d. the Mesopotamians are credited with both inventing the word and writing "Epic of Gilgamesh"

23. According to the passage, it can be understood that the word "telling" means

a. speaking

b. significant

c. soothing

d. word**y**

Questions 24 – 25 refer to the following email.

SUBJECT: MEDICAL STAFF CHANGES

To all staff:

This email is to advise you of a paper on recommended medical staff changes has been posted to the Human Resources website.

The contents are of primary interest to medical staff, other staff may be interested in reading it, particularly those in medical support roles.

The paper deals with several major issues:

1. Improving our ability to attract top quality staff to the hospital, and retain our existing staff. These changes will make our position and departmental names internationally recognizable and comparable with North American and North Asian departments and positions.

2. Improving our ability to attract top quality staff by introducing greater flexibility in the departmental structure.

3. General comments on issues to be further discussed relative to research staff.

The changes outlined in this paper are significant. I encourage you to read the document and send to me any comments you may have, so that it can be enhanced and improved.

Gordon Simms
Administrator,
Seven Oaks Regional Hospital

24. Are all hospital staff required to read the document posted to the Human Resources website?

a. Yes all staff are required to read the document.
b. No, reading the document is optional.
c. Only medical staff are required to read the document.
d. None of the above are correct.

25. Have the changes to medical staff been made?

a. Yes, the changes have been made.
b. No, the changes are only being discussed.
c. Some of the changes have been made.
d. None of the choices are correct.

Questions 26 – 30 refer to the following passage.

Passage 8 – Navy Seals

The United States Navy's Sea, Air and Land Teams, commonly known as Navy SEALs, are the U.S. Navy's principle special operations force, and a part of the Naval Special Warfare Command (NSWC) as well as the maritime component of the United States Special Operations Command (USSOCOM).

The unit's acronym ("SEAL") comes from their capacity to operate at sea, in the air, and on land – but it is their ability to work underwater that separates SEALs from most other military units in the world. Navy SEALs are trained and have been deployed in a wide variety of missions, including direct action and special reconnaissance operations, unconventional warfare, foreign internal defence, hostage rescue, counter-terrorism and other missions. All SEALs are members of either the United States Navy or the United States Coast Guard.

In the early morning of May 2, 2011 local time, a team of 40 CIA-led Navy SEALs completed an operation to kill Osama bin Laden in Abbottabad, Pakistan about 35 miles (56 km) from Islamabad, the country's capital. The Navy SEALs were part of the Naval Special Warfare Development Group, previously called "Team 6." President Barack Obama later confirmed the death of bin Laden. The unprecedented media coverage raised the public profile of the SEAL community, particularly the counter-terrorism specialists commonly known as SEAL Team 6. [13]

26. Are Navy SEALs part of USSOCOM?

a. Yes
b. No
c. Only for special operations
d. No, they are part of the US Navy

27. What separates Navy SEALs from other military units?

a. Belonging to NSWC
b. Direct action and special reconnaissance operations
c. Working underwater
d. Working for other military units in the world

28. What other military organizations do SEALs belong to?

a. The US Navy
b. The Coast Guard
c. The US Army
d. The Navy and the Coast Guard

29. What other organization participated in the Bin Laden raid?

a. The CIA
b. The US Military
c. Counter-terrorism specialists
d. None of the above

30. What is the new name for Team 6?

a. They were always called Team 6
b. The counter-terrorism specialists
c. The Naval Special Warfare Development Group
d. None of the above

Questions 31 – 33 refer to the following passage.

Passage 9 - Gardening

Gardening for food extends far into prehistory. Ornamental gardens were known in ancient times, a famous example being the Hanging Gardens of Babylon, while ancient Rome had dozens of gardens.

The earliest forms of gardens emerged from the people's need to grow herbs and vegetables. It was only later that rich individuals created gardens for purely decorative purposes.

In ancient Egypt, rich people created ornamental gardens to relax in the shade of the trees. Egyptians believed that gods liked gardens. Commonly, walls surrounded ancient Egyptian gardens with trees planted in rows.

The most popular tree species were date palms, sycamores, fig trees, nut trees, and willows. Besides ornamental gardens, wealthy Egyptians kept vineyards to produce wine.

The Assyrians are also known for their beautiful gardens in what we know today as Iraq. Assyrian gardens were very large, with some of them used for hunting and others as leisure gardens. Cypress and palm were the most popular trees in Assyrian gardens. [14]

31. Why did wealthy people in Egypt have gardens?

a. For food
b. To relax in the shade
c. For ornamentation
d. For hunting

32. What did the Egyptians believe about gardens?

a. They believed gods loved gardens.
b. They believed gods hated gardens.
c. The didn't have any beliefs about gods and Gardens.
d. They believed gods hated trees.

33. What kinds of trees did the Assyrians like?

a. The Assyrians liked date palms, sycamores, fig trees, nut trees, and willows.
b. The Assyrians liked Cypresses and palms.
c. The Assyrians didn't like trees.
d. The Assyrians liked hedges and vines.

34. Which came first, gardening for vegetables or ornamental gardens?

a. Ornamental gardens came before vegetable gardens.
b. Vegetable gardens came before ornamental gardens.
c. Vegetable and ornamental gardens appeared at the same time.
d. The passage does not give enough information.

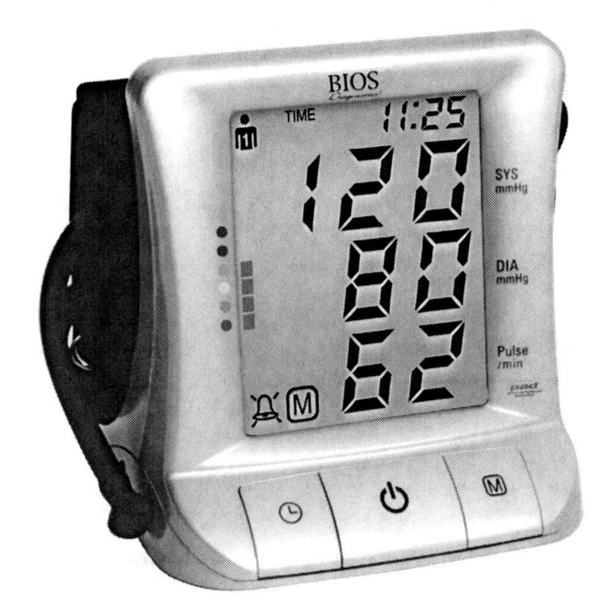

35. Consider the blood pressure gauge above. According to this gauge, what is the patient's pulse?

a. 120 beats per minute
b. 80 beats per minute
c. 62 beats per minute
d. The pulse is not shown

Questions 35 – 39 refer to the following passage.

Passage 10 - Gardens

Ancient Roman gardens are known for their statues and sculptures, which were never missing from the lives of Romans. Romans designed their gardens with hedges and vines as well as a wide variety of flowers, including acanthus, cornflowers and crocus, cyclamen, hyacinth, iris and ivy, lavender, lilies, myrtle, narcissus, poppy, rosemary and violet. Flower beds were popular in the courtyards of the rich Romans.

The Middle Ages was a period of decline in gardening. After the fall of Rome, gardening was only for growing medicinal herbs and decorating church altars.

Islamic gardens were built after the model of Persian gardens, with enclosed walls and watercourses dividing the garden into four. Commonly, the center of the garden would have a pool or pavilion. Mosaics and glazed tiles used to decorate elaborate fountains are specific to Islamic gardens. [14]

36. What is a characteristic feature of Roman gardens?

a. Statues and sculptures
b. Flower beds
c. Medicinal herbs
d. Courtyard gardens

37. When did gardening decline?

a. Before the Fall of Rome
b. Gardening did not decline
c. Before the Middle Ages
d. After the Fall of Rome

38. What kind of gardening was done during the Middle Ages?

a. Gardening with hedges and vines
b. Gardening with a wide variety of flowers
c. Gardening for herbs and church alters
d. Gardening divided by watercourses

39. What is a characteristic feature of Islamic Gardens?

a. Statues and Sculptures
b. Decorative tiles and fountains
c. Herbs
d. Flower beds

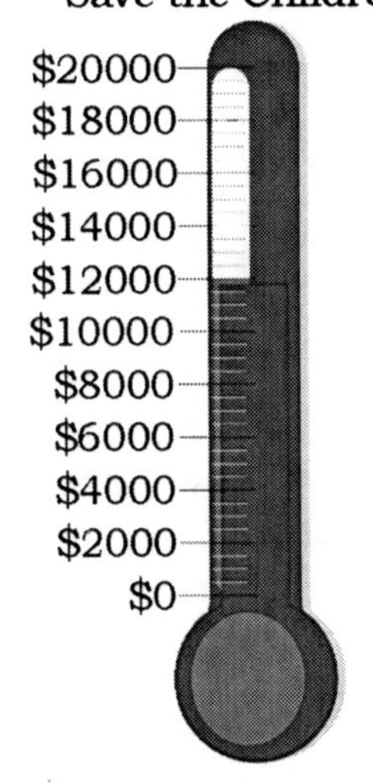

40. Consider the graphic above. The Save the Children fund has a fund-raising goal of $20,000. About how much of their goal have they achieved?

a. 3/5
b. 3/4
c. 1/2
d. 1/3

Section II – Math

1. What is 1/3 of 3/4?

a. 1/4
b. 1/3
c. 2/3
d. 3/4

2. What fraction of $1500 is $75?

a. 1/14
b. 3/5
c. 7/10
d. 1/20

3. 3.14 + 2.73 + 23.7 =

a. 28.57
b. 30.57
c. 29.56
d. 29.57

4. A woman spent 15% of her income on an item and ends with $120. What percentage of her income is left?

a. 12%
b. 85%
c. 75%
d. 95%

5. Express 0.27 + 0.33 as a fraction.

a. 3/6
b. 4/7
c. 3/5
d. 2/7

6. What is (3.13 + 7.87) X 5?

a. 65
b. 50
c. 45
d. 55

7. Reduce 2/4 X 3/4 to lowest terms.

a. 6/12
b. 3/8
c. 6/16
d. 3/4

8. 2/3 – 2/5 =

a. 4/10
b. 1/15
c. 3/7
d. 4/15

9. 2/7 + 2/3 =

a. 12/23
b. 5/10
c. 20/21
d. 6/21

10. 2/3 of 60 + 1/5 of 75 =

a. 45
b. 55
c. 15
d. 50

11. 8 is what percent of 40?

a. 10%
b. 15%
c. 20%
d. 25%

12. 9 is what percent of 36?

a. 10%
b. 15%
c. 20%
d. 25%

13. Three tenths of 90 equals:

a. 18
b. 45
c. 27
d. 36

14. .4% of 36 is

a. .144
b. 1.44
c. 14.4
d. 144

15. The physician ordered 5 mg Coumadin; 10 mg/tablet is on hand. How many tablets will you give?

a. .5 tablets
b. 1 tablet
c. .75 tablets
d. 1.5 tablets

16. The physician ordered 20 mg Tylenol/kg of body weight; on hand is 80 mg/tablet. The child weighs 12 kg. How many tablets will you give?

a. 1 tablet
b. 3 tablets
c. 2 tablets
d. 4 tablets

17. The physician ordered 20 mg Tylenol/kg of body weight; on hand is 80 mg/tablet. The child weighs 44 lb. How many tablets will you give?

a. 5 tablets
b. 5.5 tablets
c. 4.5 tablets
d. 3 tablets

18. The physician ordered 3,000 units of heparin; 5,000 U/mL is on hand. How many milliliters will you give?

a. 0.5 ml
b. 0.6 ml
c. 0.75 ml
d. 0.8 ml

19. The physician orders 60 mg Augmentin; 80 mg/mL is on hand. How many milliliters will you give?

a. 1 ml
b. 0.5 ml
c. 0.75 ml
d. 0.95 ml

20. The physician ordered 16 mg Ibuprofen/kg of body weight; on hand is 80 mg/tablet. The child weighs 15 kg. How many tablets will you give?

a. 3 tablets
b. 2 tablets
c. 1 tablet
d. 2.5 tablets

21. The physician orders 1000 mg Benbadryl liquid; 1 g/tsp is on hand. How many teaspoons will you give?

a. .75 tsp
b. 1.5 tsp
c. 1 tsp
d. 1.25 tsp

22. The physician ordered 10 units of regular insulin and 200 U/mL is on hand. How many milliliters will you give?

a. .45 ml
b. .75 ml
c. .25 ml
d. .05 ml

23. If y = 4 and x = 3, solve yx^3

a. -108
b. 108
c. 27
d. 4

24. Convert 0.007 kilograms to grams

a. 7 grams
b. 70 grams
c. 0.07 grams
d. 0.70 grams

25. Convert 16 quarts to gallons

a. 1 gallons
b. 8 gallons
c. 4 gallons
d. 4.5 gallons

26. Convert 2 teaspoons to milliliters.

a. 4.3 milliliters
b. 9 milliliters
c. 9.86 milliliters
d. 4 milliliters

27. Convert 200 meters to kilometers

a. 50 kilometers
b. 20 kilometers
c. 12 kilometers
d. 0.2 kilometers

28. Convert 72 inches to feet

a. 12 feet
b. 6 feet
c. 4 feet
d. 17 feet

29. Convert 3 yards to feet

a. 18 feet
b. 12 feet
c. 9 feet
d. 27 feet

30. Convert 45 kg. to pounds.

a. 10 pounds
b. 100 pounds
c. 1,000 pounds
d. 110 pounds

31. Convert 0.63 grams to mg.

a. 630 g.
b. 63 mg.
c. 630 mg.
d. 603 mg.

32. 5x + 3 = 7x -1. Find x

a. 1/3
b. ½
c. 1
d. 2

33. 5x+2(x+7) = 14x – 7. Find x

a. 1
b. 2
c. 3
d. 4

34. 12t -10 = 14t + 2. Find t

a. -6
b. -4
c. 4
d. 6

35. 5(z+1) = 3(z+2) + 11. Z=?

a. 2
b. 4
c. 6
d. 12

36. The price of a book went up from $20 to $25. What percent did the price increase?

a. 5%
b. 10%
c. 20%
d. 25%

37. The price of a book decreased from $25 to $20. What percent did the price decrease?

a. 5%
b. 10%
c. 20%
d. 25%

38. After taking several practice tests, Brian improved the results of his GRE test by 30%. Given that the first time he took the test Brian answered 150 questions correctly, how many questions did he answer correctly on the second test?

a. 105
b. 120
c. 180
d. 195

39. In local baseball team, 4 players (or 12.5% of the team) have long hair and the rest have short hair. How many short-haired players are there on the team?

a. 24
b. 28
c. 32
d. 50

40. In the time required to serve 43 customers, a server breaks 2 glasses and slips 5 times. The next day, the same server breaks 10 glasses. Assuming the number of glasses broken is proportional to the number of customers, how many customers did she serve?

a. 25
b. 43
c. 86
d. 215

41. A square lawn has an area of 62,500 square meters. What will the cost of building fence around it at a rate of $5.5 per meter?

a. $4000
b. $4500
c. $5000
d. $5500

42. Mr. Brown bought 5 cheese burgers, 3 drinks, and 4 fries for his family, and a cookie pack for his dog. If the price of all single items is the same at $1.30 and a 3.5% tax is added, what is the total cost of dinner for Mr. Brown?

a. $16
b. $16.9
c. $17
d. $17.5

43. The length of a rectangle is twice of its width and its area is equal to the area of a square with 12 cm. sides. What will be the perimeter of the rectangle to the nearest whole number?

a. 36 cm
b. 46 cm
c. 51 cm
d. 56 cm

44. There are 15 yellow and 35 orange balls in a basket. How many more yellow balls must be added to make the yellow balls 65%?

a. 35
b. 50
c. 65
d. 70

45. A farmer wants to plant 65,536 trees in such a way that number of rows must be equal to the number of plants in a row. How many trees should he plant in a row?

a. 1684
b. 1268
c. 668
d. 256

46. A distributor purchased 550 kilograms of potatoes for $165. He distributed these at a rate of $6.4 per 20 kilograms to 15 shops, $3.4 per 10 kilograms to 12 shops and the remainder at $1.8 per 5 kilograms. If his total distribution cost is $10, what will his profit be?

a. $10.40
b. $8.60
c. $14.90
d. $23.40

47. A farmer wants to plant trees around the outside boundaries of his rectangular field of dimensions 650 meters × 780 meters. Each tree requires 5 meters of free space all around it from the stem. How many trees can he plant?

a. 572
b. 568
c. 286
d. 282

48. A farmer wants to plant trees at the outside boundaries of his rectangular field of dimensions 650 meters × 780 meters. Each tree requires 5 meter of free space all around it from the stem. How much free area will be left?

a. 478,800 m^2
b. 492,800 m^2
c. 507,625 m^2
d. 518,256 m^2

49. How much pay does Mr. Johnson receive if he gives half of his pay to his family, $250 to his landlord, and has exactly 3/7 of his pay left over?

a. $3600
b. $3500
c. $2800
d. $1750

50. A boy has 4 red, 5 green and 2 yellow balls. He chooses two balls randomly. What is the probability that one is red and other is green?

a. 2/11
b. 19/22
c. 20/121
d. 9/11

Section III - English

1. Choose the sentence with the correct grammar.

a. Don would never have thought of that book, but you could have reminded him.

b. Don would never of thought of that book, but you could have reminded him.

c. Don would never have thought of that book, but you could of have reminded him.

d. Don would never of thought of that book, but you could of reminded him.

2. Choose the sentence with the correct grammar.

a. The mother would not of punished her daughter if she could have avoided it.

b. The mother would not have punished her daughter if she could of avoided it.

c. The mother would not of punished her daughter if she could of avoided it.

d. The mother would not have punished her daughter if she could have avoided it.

3. Choose the sentence with the correct grammar.

a. There was scarcely no food in the pantry, because nobody ate at home.

b. There was scarcely any food in the pantry, because nobody ate at home.

c. There was scarcely any food in the pantry, because not nobody ate at home.

d. There was scarcely no food in the pantry, because not nobody ate at home.

4. Choose the sentence with the correct grammar.

a. Although you may not see nobody in the dark, it does not mean that nobody is there.

b. Although you may not see anyone in the dark, it does not mean that not nobody is there.

c. Although you may not see anyone in the dark, it does not mean that no one is there.

d. Although you may not see nobody in the dark, it does not mean that not nobody is there.

5. Choose the sentence with the correct grammar.

a. Michael has lived in that house for forty years, while I has owned this one for only six weeks.

b. Michael have lived in that house for forty years, while I have owned this one for only six weeks.

c. Michael have lived in that house for forty years, while I has owned this one for only six weeks.

d. Michael has lived in that house for forty years, while I have owned this one for only six weeks.

6. Choose the sentence with the correct grammar.

a. The older children have already eat their dinner, but the baby has not yet eaten anything.

b. The older children have already eaten their dinner, but the baby has not yet ate anything.

c. The older children have already eaten their dinner, but the baby has not yet eaten anything.

d. The older children have already eat their dinner, but the baby has not yet ate anything.

7. Choose the sentence with the correct grammar.

a. If they had gone to the party, he would have gone, too.

b. If they had went to the party, he would have gone, too.

c. If they had gone to the party, he would have went, too.

d. If they had went to the party, he would have went, too.

8. Choose the sentence with the correct grammar.

a. He should have went to the appointment; instead, he went to the beach.

b. He should have gone to the appointment; instead, he went to the beach.

c. He should have went to the appointment; instead, he gone to the beach.

d. He should have gone to the appointment; instead, he gone to the beach.

9. Choose the sentence with the correct grammar.

a. Lee pronounced it's name incorrectly; it's an impatiens, not an impatience.

b. Lee pronounced its name incorrectly; its an impatiens, not an impatience.

c. Lee pronounced it's name incorrectly; its an impatiens, not an impatience.

d. Lee pronounced its name incorrectly; it's an impatiens, not an impatience.

10. Choose the sentence with the correct grammar.

a. Its important for you to know its official name; its called the Confederate Museum.

b. It's important for you to know it's official name; it's called the Confederate Museum.

c. It's important for you to know its official name; it's called the Confederate Museum.

d. Its important for you to know it's official name; it's called the Confederate Museum.

11. The Ford Motor Company was named for Henry Ford, ________.

a. which had founded the company.

b. who founded the company.

c. whose had founded the company.

d. whom had founded the company.

12. Thomas Edison ________ since he invented the light bulb, television, motion pictures, and phonograph.

a. has always been known as the greatest inventor

b. was always been known as the greatest inventor

c. must have had been always known as the greatest inventor

d. will had been known as the greatest inventor

13. The weatherman on Channel 6 said that this has been the ________.

a. most hottest summer on record

b. most hotter summer on record

c. hottest summer on record

d. hotter summer on record

14. Although Joe is tall for his age, his brother Elliot is ________ of the two.

a. the tallest

b. more tallest

c. the tall

d. the taller

15. When KISS came to town, all of the tickets _________ before I could buy one.

a. will be sold out
b. had been sold out
c. were being sold out
d. was sold out

16. The rules of most sports _________ more complicated than we often realize.

a. are
b. is
c. was
d. has been

17. Neither of the Wright Brothers _________ that they would be successful with their flying machine.

a. have any doubts
b. has any doubts
c. had any doubts
d. will have any doubts

18. The Titanic _________ mere days into its maiden voyage.

a. has already sunk
b. will already sunk
c. already sank
d. sank

19. _________ won first place in the Western Division?

a. Who
b. Whom
c. Which
d. What

20. There are now several ways to listen to music, including radio, CDs, and Mp3 files _________ you can download onto an MP3 player.

a. on which
b. who
c. whom
d. which

21. As the tallest monument in the United States, the St. Louis Arch _________.

a. has rose to an impressive 630 feet.
b. is risen to an impressive 630 feet.
c. rises to an impressive 630 feet.
d. was rose to an impressive 630 feet.

22. The tired, old woman should _________ on the sofa.

a. lie
b. lays
c. laid
d. lain

23. Did the students understand that Thanksgiving always _________ on the fourth Thursday in November?

a. fallen
b. falling
c. has fell
d. falls

24. Collecting stamps, _________ and listening to shortwave radio were Rick's main hobbies.

a. building models,
b. to build models,
c. having built models,
d. build models,

25. Choose the sentence with the correct usage.

a. The ceremony had an emotional effect on the groom, but the bride was not affected.

b. The ceremony had an emotional affect on the groom, but the bride was not affected.

c. The ceremony had an emotional effect on the groom, but the bride was not effected.

d. The ceremony had an emotional affect on the groom, but the bride was not affected.

26. Choose the sentence with the correct usage.

a. Anna was taller then Luis, but then he grew four inches in three months.

b. Anna was taller then Luis, but than he grew four inches in three months.

c. Anna was taller than Luis, but than he grew four inches in three months.

d. Anna was taller than Luis, but then he grew four inches in three months.

27. Choose the sentence with the correct usage.

a. Their second home is in Boca Raton, but there not their for most of the year.

b. They're second home is in Boca Raton, but they're not there for most of the year.

c. Their second home is in Boca Raton, but they're not there for most of the year.

d. There second home is in Boca Raton, but they're not there for most of the year.

28. Choose the sentence with the correct usage.

a. They're going to graduate in June; after that, their best option will be to go there.

b. There going to graduate in June; after that, their best option will be to go there.

c. They're going to graduate in June; after that, there best option will be to go their.

d. Their going to graduate in June; after that, their best option will be to go there

29. Choose the sentence with the correct usage.

a. You're mistaken; that is not you're book.

b. Your mistaken; that is not your book.

c. You're mistaken; that is not your book.

d. Your mistaken; that is not you're book.

30. Choose the sentence with the correct usage.

a. You're classes are on the west side of campus, but you're living on the east side.

b. Your classes are on the west side of campus, but your living on the east side.

c. Your classes are on the west side of campus, but you're living on the east side.

d. You're classes are on the west side of campus, but you're living on the east side.

31. Choose the sentence with the correct usage.

a. Disease is highly prevalent in poorer nations; the most dominant disease is malaria.

b. Disease are highly prevalent in poorer nations; the most dominant disease is malaria.

c. Disease is highly prevalent in poorer nations; the most dominant disease are malaria.

d. Disease are highly prevalent in poorer nations; the most dominant disease are malaria.

32. Choose the sentence with the correct usage.

a. Although I would prefer to have dog, I actually own a cat.

b. Although I would prefer to have a dog, I actually own cat.

c. Although I would prefer to have a dog, I actually own a cat.

d. Although I would prefer to have dog, I actually own cat.

33. Choose the sentence with the correct usage.

a. The principal of the school lived by one principle: always do your best.

b. The principle of the school lived by one principle: always do your best.

c. The principal of the school lived by one principal: always do your best.

d. The principle of the school lived by one principal: always do your best.

34. Choose the sentence with the correct usage.

a. Even with an speed limit sign clearly posted, an inattentive driver may drive too fast.

b. Even with a speed limit sign clearly posted, a inattentive driver may drive too fast.

c. Even with an speed limit sign clearly posted, a inattentive driver may drive too fast.

d. Even with a speed limit sign clearly posted, an inattentive driver may drive too fast.

35. Choose the sentence with the correct usage.

a. Except for the roses, she did not accept John's frequent gifts.
b. Accept for the roses, she did not except John's frequent gifts.
c. Accept for the roses, she did not accept John's frequent gifts.
d. Except for the roses, she did not except John's frequent gifts.

36. Choose the sentence with the correct usage.

a. Although he continued to advise me, I no longer took his advice.
b. Although he continued to advice me, I no longer took his advise.
c. Although he continued to advise me, I no longer took his advise.
d. Although he continued to advice me, I no longer took his advise.

37. Choose the sentence with the correct usage.

a. In order to adopt to the climate, we had to adopt a different style of clothing.
b. In order to adapt to the climate, we had to adapt a different style of clothing.
c. In order to adapt to the climate, we had to adopt a different style of clothing.
d. In order to adapt to the climate, we had to adapt a different style of clothing.

38. Choose the sentence with the correct usage.

a. When he's between friends, Robert seems confident, but between you and me, he is really very shy.

b. When he's among friends, Robert seems confident, but among you and me, he is really very shy.

c. When he's between friends, Robert seems confident, but among you and me, he is really very shy.

d. When he's among friends, Robert seems confident, but between you and me, he is really very shy.

39. Choose the sentence with the correct usage.

a. I will be finished at ten in the morning, and will be arriving at home at about 6:30.

b. I will be finished at about ten in the morning, and will be arriving at home at 6:30.

c. I will be finished at about ten in the morning, and will be arriving at home at about 6:30.

d. I will be finished at ten in the morning, and will be arriving at home at 6:30.

40. Choose the sentence with the correct usage.

a. Beside the red curtains and pillows, there was a red rug beside the couch.

b. Besides the red curtains and pillows, there was a red rug beside the couch.

c. Besides the red curtains and pillows, there was a red rug besides the couch.

d. Beside the red curtains and pillows, there was a red rug besides the couch.

41. Choose the sentence with the correct usage.

a. Although John can swim very well, the lifeguard may not allow him to swim in the pool.

b. Although John may swim very well, the lifeguard may not allow him to swim in the pool.

c. Although John can swim very well, the lifeguard cannot allow him to swim in the pool.

d. Although John may swim very well, the lifeguard may not allow him to swim in the pool.

42. Choose the sentence with the correct usage.

a. Her continuous absences caused a continual disruption at the office.

b. Her continual absences caused a continuous disruption at the office.

c. Her continual absences caused a continual disruption at the office.

d. Her continuous absences caused a continuous disruption at the office.

43. Choose the sentence with the correct usage.

a. During the famine, the Irish people had to emigrate to other countries; many of them immigrated to the United States.

b. During the famine, the Irish people had to immigrate to other countries; many of them immigrated to the United States.

c. During the famine, the Irish people had to emigrate to other countries; many of them emigrated to the United States.

d. During the famine, the Irish people had to immigrate to other countries; many of them emigrated to the United States.

44. Choose the sentence with the correct usage.

a. His home was farther than we expected; farther, the roads were very bad.

b. His home was farther than we expected; further, the roads were very bad.

c. His home was further than we expected; further, the roads were very bad.

d. His home was further than we expected; farther, the roads were very bad.

45. Choose the sentence with the correct usage.

a. The volunteers brought groceries and toys to the homeless shelter; the latter were given to the staff, while the former were given directly to the children.

b. The volunteers brought groceries and toys to the homeless shelter; the former was given to the staff, while the latter was given directly to the children.

c. The volunteers brought groceries and toys to the homeless shelter; the groceries were given to the staff, while the former was given directly to the children.

d. The volunteers brought groceries and toys to the homeless shelter; the latter was given to the staff, while the groceries were given directly to the children.

46. Choose the sentence with the correct usage.

a. Vegetables are a healthy food; eating them can make you more healthful.

b. Vegetables are a healthful food; eating them can make you more healthful.

c. Vegetables are a healthy food; eating them can make you more healthy.

d. Vegetables are a healthful food; eating them can make you more healthy.

47. Choose the sentence with the correct usage.

a. After you lay the books on the counter, you may lay down for a nap.

b. After you lie the books on the counter, you may lay down for a nap.

c. After you lay the books on the counter, you may lie down for a nap.

d. After you lay the books on the counter, you may lay down for a nap.

48. Choose the sentence with the correct usage.

a. After you lay the books on the counter, you may lay down for a nap.

b. After you lie the books on the counter, you may lay down for a nap.

c. After you lay the books on the counter, you may lie down for a nap.

d. After you lay the books on the counter, you may lay down for a nap.

49. Choose the sentence with the correct usage.

a. Once the chickens had layed their eggs, they lay on their nests to hatch them.

b. Once the chickens had lay their eggs, they lay on their nests to hatch them.

c. Once the chickens had laid their eggs, they lay on their nests to hatch them.

d. Once the chickens had laid their eggs, they laid on their nests to hatch them.

50. Choose the sentence with the correct usage.

a. Mrs. Foster taught me many things, but I learned the most from Mr. Wallace.

b. Mrs. Foster learned me many things, but I was taught the most by Mr. Wallace.

c. Mrs. Foster learned me many things, but I learned the most from Mr. Wallace.

d. Mrs. Foster taught me many things, but I was learned the most from Mr. Wallace.

Section IV - Critical Thinking

1. Select the option with the same relationship as fat : eat

a. walk : run

b. swim : water

c. live : breathe

d. sing : song

2. Select the option with the same relationship as dog : canine

a. porpoise : mammal

b. cat : mouse

c. tree : flower

d. elephant : large

3. Consider the following series: 23, __, 31, 37. What is the missing number?

a. 30

b. 22

c. 19

d. 29

4. Consider the following series: 3, 6, 11, 18, ... What number should come next?

a. 32

b. 29

c. 30

d. 27

5. Consider the following series: 26, 24, 20, 14, ... What number should come next?

a. 6
b. 18
c. 12
d. 8

6. Which of the following does not belong?

a. ddeeffgg
b. ffgghhii
c. nnooppqq
d. ttuuvvww

7. Which of the following does not belong?

a. 44556677
b. 33445566
c. 11223344
d. 33455666

8. Which of the following does not belong?

a. mNo
b. Stu
c. pQr
d. xYz

9. Select the option with the same relationship. Melt : Liquid Freeze : __________

a. Condense
b. Steam
c. Ice
d. Solid

10. Select the option with the same relationship. Clock : Time : : Thermometer : ____________

a. Energy
b. Radiation
c. Temperature
d. Heat

11. Select the option with the same relationship. Car : Garage : Plane : ____________

a. Harbor
b. Hanger
c. Port
d. Depot

12. Select the option with the same relationship. Acting : Theatre : : Gambling : _______________

a. Club
b. Bar
c. Casino
d. Gym

13. Consider the following series: 12, 4, 16, ___ , 36. What is the missing number?

a. 18
b. 22
c. 30
d. 20

14. Consider the following series: 3, 9, 27, ___ , 243. What is the missing number?

a. 18
b. 81
c. 39
d. 30

15. Consider the following series: 29, 39, 46, 56, ___, 25. What is the missing number?

a. 40
b. 20
c. 39
d. 15

16. Which of the following does not belong?

a. QRS
b. ACF
c. LMN
d. RST

17. Which of the following does not belong?

a. PQRs
b. aBCd
c. lMNo
d. tUVw

18. Which of the following does not belong?

a. JKLM
b. PQRS
c. ABCD
d. WXYZ

19. Select the option with the same relationship as Turntable : MP3 player

a. Horse Drawn Carriage : Car
b. Radio : Telephone
c. Calculator : Computer
d. Documentary : Movie

20. Select the option with the same relationship as Cub : Bear

a. Puppy : Dog
b. Piano : Orchestra
c. Cat : Kitten
d. Eagle : Predator

Section V – Science

1. Electricity is a general term encompassing a variety of phenomena resulting from the presence and flow of electric charge. Which of the following statements about electricity is/are true?

a. Electrically charged matter is influenced by, and produces, electromagnetic fields.

b. Electric current is a movement or flow of electrically charged particles.

c. Electric potential is a fundamental interaction between the magnetic field and the presence and motion of an electric charge.

d. An influence produced by an electric charge on other charges in its vicinity is an electric field.

2. Which of the following is/are not included in Ohm's Law?

a. Ohm's Law defines the relationships between (P) power, (E) voltage, (I) current, and (R) resistance.

b. One ohm is the resistance value through which one volt will maintain a current of one ampere.

c. Using Ohm's Law, voltage is determined using V = IR, with I equaling current and R equaling resistance.

d. An ohm (Ω) is a unit of electrical voltage.

3. The property of a conductor that restricts its internal flow of electrons is:

a. Friction

b. Power

c. Current

d. Resistance

4. In physics, ___________ is the force that opposes the relative motion of two bodies in contact.

a. Resistance

b. Abrasiveness

c. Friction

d. Antagonism

5. What is the difference, of any, between kinetic energy and potential energy?

a. Kinetic energy is the energy of a body that results from heat while potential energy is the energy possessed by an object that is chilled

b. Kinetic energy is the energy of a body that results from motion while potential energy is the energy possessed by an object by virtue of its position or state, e.g., as in a compressed spring.

c. There is no difference between kinetic and potential energy; all energy is the same.

d. Potential energy is the energy of a body that results from motion while kinetic energy is the energy possessed by an object by virtue of its position or state, e.g., as in a compressed spring.

6. What are considered the four fundamental forces of nature?

a. Gravity, electromagnetic force, weak nuclear force, and strong nuclear force

b. Gravity, electromagnetic force, negative nuclear force, and positive nuclear force

c. Polarity, electromagnetic force, weak nuclear force, and strong nuclear force

d. Gravity, chemical magnetic force, weak nuclear force, and strong nuclear force

7. Starting with the weakest, arrange the fundamental forces of nature in order of strength.

a. Gravity, Weak Nuclear Force, Electromagnetic Force, Strong Nuclear Force

b. Weak Nuclear Force, Gravity, Electromagnetic Force, Strong Nuclear Force

c. Strong Nuclear Force, Weak Nuclear Force, Electromagnetic Force, Gravity

d. Gravity, Strong Nuclear Force, Weak Nuclear Force, Electromagnetic Force

8. What is the difference between Strong Nuclear Force and Weak Nuclear Force?

a. The Strong Nuclear Force is an attractive force that binds protons and neutrons and maintains the structure of the nucleus, and the Weak Nuclear Force is responsible for the radioactive beta decay and other subatomic reactions.

b. The Strong Nuclear Force is responsible for the radioactive beta decay and other subatomic reactions, and the Weak Nuclear Force is an attractive force that binds protons and neutrons and maintains the structure of the nucleus.

c. The Weak Nuclear Force is feeble and the Strong Nuclear Force is robust.

d. The Strong Nuclear Force is a negative force that releases protons and neutrons and threatens the structure of the nucleus, and the Weak Nuclear Force is an attractive force that binds protons and neutrons and maintains the structure of the nucleus.

9. The Law of Conservation of Mass states that:

a. No detectable gain but, depending on the substances used, some loss can occur in chemical reactions.

b. No detectable gain or loss occurs in chemical reactions.

c. No detectable loss but some gain occurs in chemical reactions.

d. Depending on the substances used, substantial gain or loss can occur in chemical reactions.

10. What is the difference, if any, between convection and heat radiation?

a. Thermal radiation is the transfer of heat from one place to another by the movement of fluids; convection is electromagnetic radiation emitted from all matter due to its possessing thermal energy.

b. Convection is the transfer of heat from one place to another by the movement of fluids; thermal radiation is nuclear energy emitted from all matter due to its possessing thermal energy.

c. Convection is the transfer of heat from one place to another by the movement of fluids; thermal radiation is electromagnetic radiation emitted from all matter due to its possessing thermal energy.

d. Convection is the transfer of heat from one place to another by the movement of fluids; thermal radiation is the barely detectable light emitted from all matter due to its possessing thermal energy.

11. In ________ cells, the cell cycle is the cycle of events involving cell division, including ______, ________, and ________.

a. Prokaryotic, meiosis, cytokinesis, and interphase

b. Eukaryotic, meiosis, cytokinesis, and interphase

c. Eukaryotic, mitosis, kinematisis, and interphase

d. Eukaryotic, mitosis, cytokinesis, and interphase

12. Which, if any, of the following statements about prokaryotic cells is false?

a. Prokaryotic cells include such organisms as E. coli and Streptococcus.

b. Prokaryotic cells lack internal membranes and organelles.

c. Prokaryotic cells break down food using cellular respiration and fermentation.

d. All of these statements are true.

13. _________ is a nucleic acid that carries the genetic information in the cell and is capable of self-replication.

a. RNA
b. Triglyceride
c. DNA
d. DAR

14. The complementary bases found in DNA are ______ and _______ or _______ and ________.

a. Adenine and thymine or cytosine and guanine
b. Cytosine and thymine or adenine and guanine
c. Adenine and cytosine or thymine and guanine
d. None of the above

15. A/an _______ is the basic structural unit of nucleic acids (DNA or RNA); their sequence determines individual hereditary characteristics.

a. Gene
b. Nucleotide
c. Phosphate
d. Nitrogen base

16. _______________ is a ____________ that plays an important role in the creation of new ________.

a. Deoxyribonucleic acid (DNA) is a chain of nucleotides that plays an important role in the creation of new proteins.
b. Ribonucleic acid (RNA) is a chain of nucleotides that plays an important role in the creation of new proteins.
c. Ribonucleic acid (RNA) is a cluster of enzymes that plays an important role in the creation of new proteins.
d. Ribonucleic acid (RNA) is a chain of nucleotides that plays an important role in the creation of new genes.

17. Which, if any, of the following statements are false?

a. A mutation is a permanent change in the DNA sequence of a gene.
b. Mutations in a gene's DNA sequence can alter the amino acid sequence of the protein encoded by the gene.
c. Mutations in DNA sequences usually occur spontaneously.
d. Mutations in DNA sequences are caused by exposure to environmental agents such as sunshine.

18. ________ reactions occur in every cell and use ________ to convert glucose to energy; ________organisms such as many bacteria can release energy without the use of _________.

a. Aerobic reactions occur in every cell and use oxygen to convert glucose to energy; anaerobic organisms such as many bacteria can release energy without the use of oxygen.

b. Anaerobic reactions occur in every cell and use oxygen to convert glucose to energy; aerobic organisms such as many bacteria can release energy without the use of oxygen.

c. Aerobic reactions occur in every cell and use exercise to convert glucose to energy; anaerobic organisms such as many bacteria can release energy without the use of exercise.

d. Analogic reactions occur in every cell and use oxygen to convert glucose to energy; anaerobic organisms such as many bacteria can release energy without the use of oxygen.

19. ________ are a collection of similar cells that group together to perform a specialized function.

a. Ephithelia
b. Organs
c. Systems
d. Tissues

20. _______ tissue serves as membranes lining organs and helping to keep the body's organs separate, in place and protected; an example is the outer layer of the skin.

a. Epithelial
b. Connective
c. Nerve
d. Protein

21. Tissue that adds support and structure to the body and frequently contains fibrous strands of collagen is ________ tissue.

a. Epithelial
b. Muscle
c. Nerve
d. Connective

22. ________ tissue is a specialized tissue that can contract and contains the specialized proteins actin and myosin that slide past one another and allow movement.

a. Epithelial
b. Muscle
c. Nerve
d. Connective

23. __________ tissue contains two types of cells: neurons and glial cells and has the ability to generate and conduct electrical signals in the body.

a. Nerve
b. Connective
c. Epithelial
d. Muscle

24. A/an ________ is a group of tissues that perform a specific function or group of functions.

a. System
b. Tissue
c. Group
d. Organ

25. Among animals, examples of _______ are the heart, lungs, brain, eye, stomach, and bones; plant _____ include the roots, stems, leaves, flowers, seeds and fruits.

a. Systems
b. Organs
c. Tissues
d. Phylum

26. Our bodies have ____ different ______, including ________, ________, and ________.

a. Our bodies have 5 different systems, including circulatory, digestive, and lymphatic.

b. Our bodies have 11 different systems, including circulatory, digestive, and heart.

c. Our bodies have 11 different systems, including circulatory, digestive, and lymphatic.

d. Our bodies have 12 different systems, including circulatory, bowel, and lymphatic.

27. The _______ system absorbs excess fluid, preventing tissues from swelling, defends the body against microorganisms and harmful foreign particles, and facilitates the absorption of fat.

a. Vascular

b. Digestive

c. Circulatory

d. Lymphatic

28. The ______ system consists of _____, _____, and ______ that transport ______ to and from all tissues

a. The vascular system consists of arteries, veins, and capillaries that transport oxygen to and from all tissues.

b. The lymphatic system consists of arteries, veins, and capillaries that transport oxygen to and from all tissues.

c. The vascular system consists of arteries, stratums, and capillaries that transport oxygen to and from all tissues.

d. The vascular system consists of arteries, veins, and ducts that transport oxygen to and from all tissues.

29. What are the differences, if any, between arteries, veins, and capillaries?

a. Veins carry oxygenated blood away from the heart, arteries return oxygen-depleted blood to the heart, and capillaries are thin-walled blood vessels in which gas/ nutrient/ waste exchange occurs.

b. Capillaries carry oxygenated blood away from the heart, veins return oxygen-depleted blood to the heart, and capillaries are thin-walled blood vessels in which gas/ nutrient/ waste exchange occurs.

c. There are no differences; all perform the same function in different parts of the body.

d. Arteries carry oxygenated blood away from the heart, veins return oxygen-depleted blood to the heart, and capillaries are thin-walled blood vessels in which gas/ nutrient/ waste exchange occurs.

30. The __________ is the primary organ of the digestive tract, and may be subdivided into three segments, the _______, the _______, and the ______.

a. The stomach is the primary organ of the digestive tract, and may be subdivided into three segments, the duodenum, the jejunum, and the ileum.

b. The small intestine is the primary organ of the digestive tract, and may be subdivided into three segments, the duodenum, the jejunum, and the ileum.

c. The large intestine is the primary organ of the digestive tract, and may be subdivided into three segments, the duodenum, the jejunum, and the ileum.

d. The small intestine is the primary organ of the digestive tract, and may be subdivided into three segments, the duodenum, the jejunum, and the ilex.

31. The ______system defends our bodies against infections and disease through three types of response systems: the _______ response, the ________ response, and the ______ response.

a. The vascular system defends our bodies against infections and disease through three types of response systems: the anatomic response, the inflammatory response, and the immune response.

b. The immune system defends our bodies against infections and disease through three types of response systems: the anatomic response, the inflammatory response, and the immune response.

c. The immune system defends our bodies against infections and disease through three types of response systems: the automatic response, the flammatory response, and the immune response.

d. The epithelial system defends our bodies against infections and disease through three types of response systems: the anatomic response, the inflammatory response, and the immune response.

32. The _____________ system is composed of all of the bones, cartilage, muscles, joints, tendons and ligaments in a person's body.

a. Musculoskeletal

b. Muscular

c. Skeletal

d. Connective

33. The _____________ is a muscular tube lined by a special layer of cells, called _______; its primary purpose is to break food down into ______, which can be absorbed into the body to provide energy.

a. The epithelium tract is a muscular tube lined by a special layer of cells, called gastric; its primary purpose is to break food down into nutrients, which can be absorbed into the body to provide energy.

b. The gastrointestinal tract is a muscular tube lined by a special layer of cells, called ileum; its primary purpose is to break food down into oxygen, which can be absorbed into the body to provide energy.

c. The gastrointestinal tract is a muscular tube lined by a special layer of cells, called epithelium; its primary purpose is to break food down into nutrients, which can be absorbed into the body to provide energy.

d. The esophageal tract is a muscular tube lined by a special layer of cells, called epithelium; its primary purpose is to break food down into nutrients, which can be absorbed into the body to provide energy.

34. The ______________ states that, in a chemical change, _______ can be neither _____ nor _______, but only changed from _____________.

a. The Law of the Preservation of Matter states that, in a chemical change, energy can be neither created nor destroyed, but only changed from one form to another.

b. The Law of the Conservation of Energy states that, in a chemical change, energy can be neither created nor destroyed, but only changed from one atomic number to another.

c. The Law of the Conservation of Energy states that, in a chemical change, energy can be neither created nor destroyed, but only changed from one form to another.

d. The Law of the Conservation of Energy states that, in a chemical change, energy can be neither duplicated nor destroyed, but only changed from one form to another.

35. A ________ is a process that transforms one set of chemical substances to another; the substances used are known as _______ and those formed are ________.

a. A chemical change is a process that transforms one set of chemical substances to another; the substances used are known as products and those formed are reactants.

b. A biological change is a process that transforms one set of chemical substances to another; the substances used are known as reactants and those formed are products.

c. A chemical change is a process that transforms one set of chemical substances to another; the substances used are known as reactants and those formed are products.

d. A chemical variation is a process that transforms one set of chemical substances to another; the substances used are known as reactants and those formed are products.

36. ________ is the most abundant element in the Earth's crust and appears on the Atomic Table as the letter ____.

a. Nitrogen, N

b. Oxygen, O

c. Silicon, Si

d. Sodium, Na

37. _______ is the series of chemical reactions resulting in the _____ of organic compounds, and _______ is the series of chemical reactions that _______ larger molecules.

a. Anabolism is the series of chemical reactions resulting in the synthesis of inorganic compounds, and catabolism is a series of chemical reactions that break down larger molecules.

b. Anabolism is the series of chemical reactions resulting in the synthesis of organic compounds, and catabolism is a series of chemical reactions that combine larger molecules.

c. Catabolism is the series of chemical reactions resulting in the synthesis of organic compounds, and anabolism is a series of chemical reactions that break down larger molecules.

d. Anabolism is the series of chemical reactions resulting in the synthesis of organic compounds, and catabolism is a series of chemical reactions that break down larger molecules.

38. A(n) ______ is a chemical involved in, but not changed by, a chemical reaction by which chemical bonds are _______ and reactions __________.

a. A propellant is a chemical involved in, but not changed by, a chemical reaction by which chemical bonds are weakened and reactions accelerated.

b. A reagent is a chemical involved in, but not changed by, a chemical reaction by which chemical bonds are strengthened and reactions accelerated.

c. A catalyst is a chemical involved in, but not changed by, a chemical reaction by which chemical bonds are weakened and reactions slowed.

d. A catalyst is a chemical involved in, but not changed by, a chemical reaction by which chemical bonds are weakened and reactions accelerated.

39. ________________ states that when two elements combine with each other to form more than one compound, the weights of one element that combine with a fixed weight of the other are in a ratio of small whole numbers.

a. The Law of Multiple Proportions

b. The Law of Definite Proportions

c. The Law of the Conservation of Energy

d. The Law of Averages

40. ________________ stats that every chemical compound contains fixed and constant proportions (by weight) of its constituent elements.

a. The Law of Multiple Proportions

b. The Law of the Preservation of Matter

c. The Law of the Conservation of Energy

d. The Law of Definite Proportions

41. __________ states that, in a given _____, _________ can have the __________.

a. The Law of Definite Proportions states that, in a given atom, no two electrons can have the same set of four quantum numbers.

b. The Pauli Exclusion Principle states that, in a given atom, no four electrons can have the same set of two quantum numbers.

c. The Pauli Exclusion Principle states that, in a given molecule, no two electrons can have a different set of four quantum numbers.

d. The Pauli Exclusion Principle states that, in a given atom, no two electrons can have the same set of four quantum numbers.

42. According to the tenets of Dalton's atomic theory, which of the following is true:

a. All matter is made up of tiny, interconnected particles called atoms.

b. All atoms of an element are alike in weight, and this weight is specific to the kind of atom.

c. Atoms can be subdivided, created, or destroyed.

d. In chemical reactions, atoms are not combined, separated, or rearranged.

43. Atoms of _________ __________ combine in _______ _______ ratios to form chemical _______.

a. Atoms of different elements combine in simple whole-number ratios to form chemical compounds.

b. Atoms of different components combine in simple fractional ratios to form chemical compounds.

c. Atoms of the same element combine in simple whole-number ratios to form chemical compounds.

d. Atoms of different elements combine in simple whole-number ratios to form chemical mixtures.

44. Which of the following statements about the periodic table of the elements are true?

a. On the periodic table, the elements are arranged according to their atomic mass.

b. The way in which the elements are arranged allows for predictions about their behavior.

c. The vertical columns of the table are called rows.

d. The horizontal rows of the table are called groups.

45. __________ _______ is the minimum amount of energy required to remove an electron from an atom or ion in the gas phase.

a. Ionization energy
b. Valence energy
c. Atomic energy
d. Ionic energy

46. A(an) ________ _________ is one half the distance between nuclei of atoms of the same element, when the atoms are bound by a single covalent bond or are in a metallic crystal.

a. Ionic radius
b. Metallic radius
c. Covalent radius
d. Atomic radius

47. What are the differences, if any, between anions and cations?

a. An anion is a negatively charged ion, and a cation is a positively charged ion.
b. Anions are typically formed by nonmetals, and metals usually form cations.
c. A & B
d. None of the Above

48. The radius of atoms obtained from ________ bond lengths is called the _______ radius; the radius from interatomic distances in metallic crystals is called the _______ radius.

a. The radius of atoms obtained from valent bond lengths is called the valent radius; the radius from interatomic distances in metallic crystals is called the metallic radius.

b. The radius of atoms obtained from covalent bond lengths is called the covalent radius; the radius from interatomic distances in nonmetallic crystals is called the nonmetallic radius.

c. The radius of atoms obtained from covalent bond lengths is called the covalent radius; the radius from interatomic distances in metallic crystals is called the metallic radius.

d. The radius of atoms obtained from covalent bond lengths is called the covalent radius; the radius from interatomic distances in ionic crystals is called the ionic radius.

49. A(an) _______ _______ is a regular variation in element properties with _______ atomic number that is ultimately due to _______ variations in atomic structure.

a. A episodic trend is a regular variation in element properties with increasing atomic number that is ultimately due to regular variations in atomic structure.

b. A periodic trend is a regular variation in element properties with decreasing atomic number that is ultimately due to regular variations in atomic structure.

c. A periodic trend is a regular variation in element properties with increasing atomic number that is ultimately due to irregular variations in atomic structure.

d. A periodic trend is a regular variation in element properties with increasing atomic number that is ultimately due to regular variations in atomic structure.

50. Which of the following statements about nonmetals are false?

a. A nonmetal is a substance that conducts heat and electricity poorly

b. The majority of the known chemical elements are nonmetals

c. A nonmetal is brittle or waxy or gaseous

d. All of the above are true

Answer Key

Section 1 – Reading

1. B
We can infer from this passage that sickness from an infectious disease can be easily transmitted from one person to another.

From the passage, "Infectious pathologies are also called communicable diseases or transmissible diseases, due to their potential of transmission from one person or species to another by a replicating agent (as opposed to a toxin)."

2. A
Two other names for infectious pathologies are communicable diseases and transmissible diseases.

From the passage, "Infectious pathologies are also called communicable diseases or transmissible diseases, due to their potential of transmission from one person or species to another by a replicating agent (as opposed to a toxin)."

3. C
Infectivity describes the ability of an organism to enter, survive and multiply in the host. This is taken directly from the passage, and is a definition type question.

Definition type questions can be answered quickly and easily by scanning the passage for the word you are asked to define.

"Infectivity" is an unusual word, so it is quick and easy to scan the passage looking for this word.

4. B
We know an infection is not synonymous with an infectious disease because an infection may not cause important clinical symptoms or impair host function.

5. A
Low blood sugar occurs both in diabetics and healthy adults.

6. B
None of the statements are the author's opinion.

7. A
The author's purpose is to inform.

8. A
The only statement that is **not** a detail is, "A doctor can diagnosis this medical condition by asking the patient questions and testing."

9. C
The cumulus stage of a thunderstorm is the beginning of the thunderstorm.

This is taken directly from the passage, "The first stage of a thunderstorm is the cumulus, or developing stage."

10. D
The passage lists four ways that air is heated. One way is, heat created by water vapor condensing into liquid.

11. A
The sequence of events can be taken from these sentences:

As the moisture carried by the [1] air currents rises, it rapidly cools into liquid drops of water, which appear as cumulus clouds. As the water vapor condenses into liquid, it [2] releases heat, which warms the air. This in turn causes the air to become less dense than the surrounding dry air and [3] rise farther.

12. C
This question tests the reader's vocabulary skills. The uses of the negatives "but" and "less," especially right next to each other, may confuse readers into answer-

ing with options A or D, which list words that are the opposite of "militant." Readers may also be confused by the comparison of healthy people with what is being described as an overly healthy person -- both people are good, but the reader may look for which one is "worse" in the comparison, and therefore stray toward the opposite words.

One key to understanding the meaning of "militant" is to look at the root; and then easily associate it with "military" and gain a sense of what the word signifies: defense (especially considered that the immune system defends the body). Option C is correct over B because "militant" is an adjective, just as the words in C are, whereas the words in option B are nouns.

13. C
This question tests the reader's understanding of function within writing. The other options are all details included surrounding the quoted text, and may therefore confuse the reader. Option A somewhat contradicts what is said earlier in the paragraph, which is that tests and treatments are improving, and probably doctors are along with them, but the paragraph doesn't actually mention doctors, and the subject of the question is the medicine. Option B may seem correct to readers who aren't careful to understand that, while the author does mention the large number of people affected, the author is touching on the realities of living with allergies rather about the likelihood of curing all allergies. Similarly, while the the author does mention the "balance" of the body, which is easily associated with "wholesome," the author is not really making an argument and especially is not making an extreme statement that allergy medicines should be outlawed. Again, because the article's tone is on living with allergies, option C is an appropriate choice that fits with the title and content of the text.

14. B
This question tests the reader's inference skills. The text does not state who is doing the recommending, but the use of the "patients," as well as the general context of the passage, lends itself to the logical partner, "doctors," option B.

The author does mention the recommendation but doesn't present it as her own (i.e. "I recommend that"), so option A may be eliminated. It may seem plausible that people with allergies (option D) may recommend medicines or products to other people with allergies, but the text does not necessarily support this interaction taking place. Option C may be selected because the EpiPen is specifically mentioned, but the use of the phrase "such as" when it is introduced is not limiting enough to assume the recommendation is coming from its creators.

15. C
You would find information about natural selection and adaptation in the ecology section which begins on page 110.

16. D
Clouds on Earth are made of water droplets or ice crystals. Clouds in space are made of different materials attracted by gravity.

Choice D is the best answer. Notice also that Choice D is the most specific.

17. C
The main idea is the first sentence of the passage; a cloud is a visible mass of droplets or frozen crystals floating in the atmosphere above the surface of the Earth or other planetary body.

The main idea is very often the first sentence of the paragraph.

18. C
Nephology, which is the study of cloud physics.

19. C
This question asks about the process, and gives options that can be confirmed or eliminated easily.

From the passage, "Dense, deep clouds reflect most light, so they appear white, at least from the top. Cloud droplets scatter light very efficiently, so the farther into a cloud light travels, the weaker it gets. This accounts for the gray or dark appearance at the base of large clouds."

We can eliminate option A, since water droplets inside the cloud do not reflect light is false.

We can eliminate option B, since, water droplets outside the cloud reflect light, it appears dark, is false.

Option C is correct.

20. C
This question tests the reader's summarizing skills. The use of the word "actually" in describing what kind of people poets are, as well as other moments like this, may lead readers to selecting options B or D, but the author is more information than trying to persuade readers. The author gives no indication that she loves poetry (B) or that people, students specifically (D), should write poems. Option A is incorrect because the style and content of this paragraph do not match those of a foreword; forewords usually focus on the history or ideas of a specific poem in order to introduce it more fully and help it stand out against other poems. The author here focuses on several poems and gives broad statements. Instead, she tells a kind of story about poems, giving three very broad time periods in which to discuss them, thereby giving a brief history of poetry, as option C states.

21. A
This question tests the reader's summarizing skills. Key words in the topic sentences of each of the paragraphs ("oldest," "Renaissance," "modern") should give the reader an idea that the author is moving chronologically. The opening and closing sentence-paragraphs are broad and talk generally. Option B seems reasonable, but epic poems are mentioned in two paragraphs, eliminating the idea that only new types of poems are used in each paragraph. Option C is also easily eliminated because the author clearly mentions several different poets, groups of people, and poems. Option D also seems reasonable, considering that the author does move from older forms of poetry to newer forms, but use of "so (that)" makes this statement false, for the author gives no indication that she is rushing (the paragraphs are about the same size) or that she prefers modern poetry.

22. D
This question tests the reader's attention to detail. The key word is "invented"--it ties together the Mesopotamians, who invented the written word, and the fact that they, as the inventors, also invented and used poetry. The other selections focus on other details mentioned in the passage, such as that the Renaissance's admiration of the Greeks (C) and that Beowulf is in Old English (A). Option B may seem like an attractive answer because it is unlike the others and because the idea of heroes seems rooted in ancient and early civilizations.

23. B
This question tests the reader's vocabulary and contextualization skills. "Telling" is not an unusual word, but it may be used here in a way that is not familiar to readers, as an adjective rather than a verb in gerund form. Option A may seem like the obvious answer to a reader looking for a verb to match the use they are familiar with. If the reader understands that the word is being used as an adjective and that A is a ploy, they may opt to select

option D, "wordy," but it does not make sense in context. Option C can be easily eliminated, and doesn't have any connection to the paragraph or passage. "Significant" (B) does make sense contextually, especially relative to the phrase "give insight" used later in the sentence.

24. B
Reading the document posted to the Human Resources website is optional.

25. B
The document is recommended changes and have not be implemented yet.

26. A
Navy SEALS are the maritime component of the United States Special Operations Command (USSOCOM).

27. C
Working underwater separates SEALs from other military units. This is taken directly from the passage.

28. D
SEALs also belong to the Navy and the Coast Guard.

29. A
The CIA also participated. From the passage, the raid was conducted by a "team of 40 *CIA-led* Navy SEALS."

30. C
From the passage, "The Navy SEALs were part of the Naval Special Warfare Development Group, previously called 'Team 6.' "

31. B
This question is taken directly from the passage. Scan the passage for the word "Egypt" to find the answer quickly.

32. A
The Egyptians believed gods loved gardens.

33. B
Cypresses and palms were the most popular trees in Assyrian Gardens.

34. B
Vegetable gardens came before ornamental gardens.

The earliest forms of gardens emerged from the people's need to grow herbs and vegetables. It was only later that rich individuals created gardens for the purely decorative purpose.

35. C
According to the blood pressure gauge, the patient's pulse is 62 beats per minute.

36. A
The ancient Roman gardens are known by their statues and sculptures ... from the first sentence.

37. D
After the fall of Rome, gardening was only for medicinal purposes, AND gardening declined in the Middle Ages, so we can infer gardening declined after the fall of Rome.

38. C
From the passage, "After the fall of Rome gardening was only done with the purpose of growing medicinal herbs and decorating church altars," so Choice C.

39. B
From the passage, "Mosaics and glazed tiles used to decorate elaborate fountains are specific to Islamic gardens."

40. A
The Save the Children's fund has raised $12,000 out of $20,000, or 12/20. Simplifying, 12/20 = 3/5

Section II – Math Answer Key

1. A
1/3 X 3/4 = 3/12 = 1/4
2. D
75/1500 = 15/300 = 3/60 = 1/20

3. D
3.14 + 2.73 = 5.87 and 5.87 + 23.7 = 29.57

4. B
Spent 15% - 100% - 15% = 85%

5. C
To convert a decimal to a fraction, take the places of decimal as your denominator, here 2, so in 0.27, '7' is in the 100th place, so the fraction is 27/100 and 0.33 becomes 33/100.

Next estimate the answer quickly to eliminate obvious wrong choices. 27/100 is about 1/4 and 33/100 is 1/3. 1/3 is slightly larger than 1/4, and 1/4 + 1/4 is 1/2, so the answer will be slightly larger than 1/2.

Looking at the choices, Choice A can be eliminated since 3/6 = 1/2. Choice D, 2/7 is less than 1/2 and can also be eliminated. So the answer is going to be Choice B or Choice C.

Do the calculation, 0.27 + 0.33 = 0.60 and 0.60 = 60/100 = 3/5, Choice C is correct.

6. D
3.13 + 7.87 = 11 and 11 X 5 = 55

7. B
2/4 X 3/4 = 6/16, and lowest terms = 3/8

8. D
2/3-2/5 = 10-6 /15 = 4/15

9. C
2/7 + 2/3 = 6+14 /21 (21 is the common denominator) = 20/21

10. B
2/3 x 60 = 40 and 1.5 x 75 = 15, 40 + 15 = 55

11. C
This is an easy question, and shows how you can solve some questions without doing the calculations. The question is, 8 is what percent of 40. Take easy percentages for an approximate answer and see what you get.

10% is easy to calculate because you can drop the zero, or move the decimal point. 10% of 40 = 4, and 8 = 2 X 4, so, 8 must be 2 X 10% = 20%.

Here are the calculations which confirm the quick approximation.
8/40 = X/100 = 8 * 100 / 40X = 800/40 = X = 20

12. D
This is the same type of question which illustrates another method to solve quickly without doing the calculations. The question is, 9 is what percent of 36?

Ask, what is the relationship between 9 and 36? 9 X 4 = 36 so they are related by a factor of 4. If 9 is related to 36 by a factor of 4, then what is related to 100 (to get a percent) by a factor of 4?

To visualize:

9 X 4 = 36
Z X 4 = 100

So the answer is 25. 9 has the same relation to 36 as 25 has to 100.

Here are the calculations which confirm the quick approximation.
9/36 = X/100 = 9 * 100 / 36X = 900/36

= 25

13. C
3/10 * 90 = 3 * 90/10 = 27

14. A
.4/100 * 36 = .4 * 36/100 = .144

15. A
5 mg/10/mg X 1 tab/1 = .5 tablets

16. B
Step 1: Set up the formula to calculate the dose to be given in mg as per weight of the child:-
Dose ordered X Weight in Kg = Dose to be given
Step 2: 20 mg X 12 kg = 240 mg
240 mg/80 mg X 1 tab/1 = 240/80 = 3 tablets

17. A
Set up the formula to calculate the dose to be given in mg as per weight of the child:-
Dose ordered X Weight in Kg = Dose to be given
Step 2: 20 mg X 20 kg = 400 mg (Convert 44 lb to Kg, 1 lb = 0.4536 kg, hence 44 lb = 19.95 kg approx. 20 kg)
400 mg/80 mg X 1 tab/1 = 400/80 = 5 tablets

18. B
3000 units/5000 units X 1 ml/1 = 3000/5000 = 0.6 ml

19. C
60 mg/80 mg X 1 ml/1 = 60/80 = 0.75 ml

20. A
Dose ordered X Weight in Kg = Dose to be given
16 mg X 15 kg = 240 mg
240 mg/80 mg X 1 tab/1 = 240/80 = 3 tablets

21. C
(Convert 1 g = 1000 mg)
1000 mg/1000 mg X 1 tsp/1 = 1000/1000 = 1 tsp

22. D
10 units/200 units X 1 ml/1 = 10/200 = 0.05 ml

23. B
$(4)(3)^3 = (4)(27) = 108$

24. A
1000g = 1kg., 0.007 = 1000 x 0.007 = 7g.

25. C
4 quarts = 1 gallon, 16 quarts = 16/4 = 4 gallons

26. C
1 teaspoon = 4.93 milliliters (U.S.), 2 tp = 4.93 x 2 = 9.86 ml.

27. D
1,000 meters = 1 kilometer, 200 m = 200/1,000 = 0.2 km.

28. B
12 inches = 1 ft., 72 inches = 72/12 = 6 feet

29. C
1 yard = 3 feet, 3 yards = 3 feet x 3 = 9 feet

30. B
0.45 kg = 1 pound, 1 kg. = 1/0.45 and 45 kg = 1/0.45 x 45 = 99.208, or 100 pounds

31. C
1 g = 1,000 mg. 0.63 g = 0.63 x 1,000 = 630 mg.

32. D
To solve for x,
5x – 7x + 3 = -1
5x – 7x = -1 -3
-2x = -4
x = -4/ -2
x = 2

33. C
To solve for x, first simplify the equation
5x + 2x + 14 = 14x – 7
7x + 14 = 4x -7

7x – 14x + 14 = -7
7x – 14x = -7 – 14
-7x = -21
x = -21/-7
x=3

34. A
5z + 5 = 3z +6 + 11
5z -3z + 5 =6 + 11
5z – 3z = 6 + 11 -5
2z = 17 – 5
2z = 12
z= 12/2
z= 6

35. C
5z + 5 = 3z +6 + 11
5z -3z + 5 =6 + 11
5z – 3z = 6 + 11 -5
2z = 17 – 5
2z = 12
z= 12/2
z= 6

36. D
Price increased by \$5 (\$25-\$20). The percent increase is 5/20 x 100 = 5 x 5=25%

37. C
Price decreased by \$5 (\$25-\$20). The percent increase = 5/25 x 100 = 5 x 4 =20%

38. D
30/100 x 150 = 3 x 15 = 45 (increase in number of correct answers). So the number of correct answers in second test = 150 + 45 = 195

39. B
Let total number of players= X
Let the number of players with long hair=Y and the number of players with short hair=Z
Then X = 4+Z
Y= 12% of X
Z= X - 4
12.5% of X = 4
Converting from decimal to fraction gives 12.5%=125/10 x 1/100=125/1000, therefore 12.5% of =125/1000X=4
Solve for X by multiplying both sides by 1000/125, X=4 x 1000/125=32
Z = x – 4
Z = 32 – 4
z or number of short haired players = 28

40. D
2 glasses are broken for 43 customers so 1 glass breaks for every 43/2 customers served, therefore 10 glasses implies 43/2 x 10=215

41. D
As the lawn is square , the length of one side will be the square root of the area. √62,500 = 250 meters. So, the perimeter is found by 4 times the length of the side of the square:

250•4 = 1000 meters.

Since each meter costs \$5.5, the total cost of the fence will be 1000•5.5 = \$5,500.

42. D
The price of all the single items is same and there are 13 total items. So the total cost will be 13 × 1.3 = \$16.9. After 3.5 percent tax this amount will become 16.9 × 1.035 = \$17.5.

43. C
Area of the square = 12 × 12 = 144 cm^2
Let x be the width, then 2x be the length of rectangle, so its area will be $2x^2$ and perimeter will be 2(2x+x)=6x
According to the condition
$2x^2 = 144$
X = 8.48 cm
The perimeter will be
Perimeter=6×8.48
=50.88
=51 cm.

44. B
There are 50 balls in the basket now. Let x be the number of yellow balls to be added to make 65%. So the equation becomes

X + 15 /X + 50 = 65/100
X = 50

45. D
Let x be number of rows, and number of trees in a row. So equation becomes
$X^2 = 65536$
$X = 256$

46. B
The distribution is done in three different rates and amounts:

\$6.4 per 20 kilograms to 15 shops ...
20•15 = 300 kilograms distributed

\$3.4 per 10 kilograms to 12 shops ...
10•12 = 120 kilograms distributed

550 - (300 + 120) = 550 - 420 = 130 kilograms left. This amount is distributed by 5 kilogram portions. So, this means that there are 130/5 = 26 shops.

\$1.8 per 130 kilograms.

We need to find the amount he earned overall these distributions.

\$6.4 per 20 kilograms : 6.4•15 = \$96 for 300 kilograms

\$3.4 per 10 kilograms : 3.4•12 = \$40.8 for 120 kilograms

\$1.8 per 5 kilograms : 1.8•26 = \$46.8 for 130 kilograms

So, he earned 96 + 40.8 + 46.8 = \$ 183.6

The total distribution cost is given as \$10

The profit is found by: Money earned - money spent ... It is important to remember that he bought 550 kilograms of potatoes for \$165 at the beginning:

Profit = 183.6 - 10 - 165 = \$8.6

47. D
Each tree will require a 10-meter diametric space around its stem. So 65 trees can be planted along 650-meter side. Similarly, 65 along the other side. However, along the 780 meter side, the first tree will be after 10 meters at both edges, so 76 trees can be planted long that side.

Total number of trees then will be
65×2+76×2=282

48. A
As one tree requires 10-meter diametric space, or, a 10-meter space on all four sides will be left. Therefore, the dimensions left are 630×760=478,800 m^2.

49. B
We check the fractions taking place in the question. We see that there is a "half" (that is 1/2) and 3/7. So, we multiply the denominators of these fractions to decide how to name the total money. We say that Mr. Johnson has 14x at the beginning; he gives half of this, meaning 7x, to his family. \$250 to his landlord. He has 3/7 of his money left. 3/7 of 14x is equal to:

14x•(3/7) = 6x

So,

Spent money is: 7x + 250

Unspent money is: 6x

Total money is: 14x

We write an equation: total money = spent money + unspent money

14x = 7x + 250 + 6x

14x - 7x - 6x = 250

x = 250

We are asked to find the total money that is 14x:

14x = 14•250 = \$3500

50. A
The probability that the 1st ball drawn is red = 4/11
The probability that the 2nd ball drawn is green = 5/10
The combined probability will then be
4/11 X 5/10 = 20/110 = 2/11

Section III English

1. A
The third conditional is used for talking about an unreal situation (a situation that did not happen) in the past. For example, "If I had studied harder, [if clause] I would have passed the exam" [main clause]. This has the same meaning as, "I failed the exam, because I didn't study hard enough."

2. D
The third conditional is used for talking about an unreal situation (a situation that did not happen) in the past. For example, "If I had studied harder, [if clause] I would have passed the exam" [main clause]. This has the same meaning as, "I failed the exam, because I didn't study hard enough."

3. B
In double negative sentences, one negative is replaced with "any."

4. C
In double negative sentences, one negative is replaced with "any."

5. D
The present perfect tense cannot be used with specific time expressions such as yesterday, one year ago, last week, when I was a child, at that moment, that day, one day, etc. The present perfect tense is used with unspecific expressions such as ever, never, once, many times, several times, before, so far, already, yet, etc.

6. C
The present perfect tense cannot be used with specific time expressions such as yesterday, one year ago, last week, when I was a child, at that moment, that day, one day, etc. The present perfect tense is used with unspecific expressions such as ever, never, once, many times, several times, before, so far, already, yet, etc.

7. A
"Went" is used in the simple past tense. "Gone" is used in the past perfect tense.

8. B
"Went" is used in the simple past tense. "Gone" is used in the past perfect tense.

9. D
"It's" is a contraction for it is or it has. "Its" is a possessive pronoun.

10. C
"It's" is a contraction for it is or it has. "Its" is a possessive pronoun.

11. B
The sentence refers to a person, so "who" is the only correct option.

12. A
The sentence requires the past perfect "has always been known." Furthermore, this is the only grammatically correct choice.

13. C
The superlative, "hottest," is used when expressing a temperature greater than that of anything to which it is being compared.

14. D
When comparing two items, use "the taller." When comparing more than two items, use "the tallest."

15. B
The past perfect form is used to describe an event that occurred in the past and

prior to another event. Here there are two things that happened, both of them in the past, and something the person wanted to do.

Event 1: Kiss came to town
Event 2: All the tickets sold out
What I wanted to do: Buy a ticket

The events are arranged:

When KISS came to town, all the tickets had been sold out before I could buy one.

16. A
The subject is "rules" so the present tense plural form, "are," is used to agree with "realize."

17. C
The simple past tense, "had," is correct because it refers to completed action in the past.

18. D
The simple past tense, "sank," is correct because it refers to completed action in the past.

19. A
"Who" is correct because the question uses an active construction. "To whom was first place given?" is passive construction.

20. D
"Which" is correct, because the files are objects and not people.

21. C
The simple present tense, "rises," is correct.

22. A
"Lie" does not require a direct object, while "lay" does. The old woman might lie on the couch, which has no direct object, or she might lay the book down, which has the direct object, "the book."

23. D
The simple present tense, "falls," is correct because it is repeated action.

24. A
The present progressive, "building models," is correct in this sentence; it is required to match the other present progressive verbs.

25. A
"Affect" is a verb, while "effect" is a noun.

26. D
"Than" is used for comparison. "Then" is used to indicate a point in time.

27. C
"There" indicates a state of existence. "Their" is used for third person plural possession. "They're" is the contracted form of "they are."

28. A
"There" indicates a state of existence. "Their" is used for third person plural possession. "They're" is the contraction of "they are."

29. C
"Your" is the possessive form of "you." "You're" is the contraction of "you are."

30. C
"Your" is the possessive form of "you." "You're" is the contraction of "you are."

31. A
Disease is a singular noun.

32. C
Both "dog" and "cat" in this sentence are singular nouns and require the article "a."

33. A
The word "principal" is a synonym for primary or major. "Principle" means a fundamental truth.

34. D
The article "a" come before a noun that begins with a consonant, while "an" comes before a noun that begins with a vowel.

35. A
"Except" means to exclude something. "Accept" means to receive something, or to agree to an idea.

36. A
"Advise" is a verb that means to offer advice, which is a noun.

37. C
"Adapt" means to change or accommodate. "Adopt" means to accept, embrace, or to assume responsibility or ownership for something or someone.

38. D
"Among" is used with more than two items, while "between" is limited to two items.

39. D
"At" refers to a specific time or location, while "about" is approximate.

40. B
"Beside" means next to, and "besides" means in addition to.

41. A
"Can" is used when describing ability or capability. "May" is a request or the granting of permission.

42. B
"Continuous" means a time period without interruption, or ongoing. "Continual" is used for actions that are frequent and repetitive, or that continue almost without interruption.

43. A
"Emigrate" means to leave one's country, usually in order to immigrate to another country to live.

44. A
"Farther" is reserved for physical distance, and "further" is used for figurative distance, or to mean "in addition."

45. B
"Former" refers to the first of two things; "latter" to the second of two things.

46. D
"Healthy" describes people or animals that are in good health. "Healthful" is generally used in formal speech or writing, and refers to things that are good for health.

47. C
"Lie" does not require a direct object, while "lay" does. In this sentence, "lay" is followed by the direct object, "the books."

48. C
"Lie" does not require a direct object, while "lay" does. In this sentence, "lay" is followed by the direct object, "the books."

49. C
This is the correct choice.

50. B
"Learn" means to receive and integrate knowledge or an experience. "Teach" means to impart knowledge to another.

Section IV - Critical Thinking

1. C
This is a cause and effect relationship. You must eat to become fat, in the same way you must breathe to live.

2. A
This is a definition relationship. A dog is a canine in the same way a porpoise is a mammal.

3. D
The numbers are primes (divisible only by 1 and themselves).

4. D
The interval, beginning with 3, increases by 2 each time. So, 3 + 3 = 6, 6 + 5 = 11, 11 + 7 = 18, 18 + 9 = 27.

5. A
The interval, beginning with 2, increases by 2 each time and is subtracted from the previous number. So, 26 - 2 = 24, 24 - 4 = 20, 20 - 6 = 14.

6. B
This is a vowel and consonant relationship. All of the choices have vowels in positions 3 and 4.

7. D
This is a repetition patter All of the choices have consecutive numbers repeated twice.

8. B
This is a capital small letter relationship. All choices have the middle letter capitalized.

9. D
This is a process relationship. The first word is the process which creates the second. for example, ice melts to liquid in the same way water freezes to create a solid.

10. C
This is a measurement relationship. Clocks measure time in the same way thermometers measure temperature.

11. B
A car is kept in a garage the same way a plane is kept in a hangar.

12. C
This is a place relationship. Acting is done in a theatre in the same way gambling is done in a casino.

13. D
Each number is the sum of the previous two numbers.

14. B
The number triples each time.

15. D
Each number is ten less than the next number. E.g.. 29 is 10 less than 39.

16. B
ACF is not a sequence of consecutive letters.

17. A
Capital small letter relationship. All choices have the middle two letters capitalized except Choice A.

18. C
This is a vowel and consonant relationship. All of the choices except Choice C, are consonants.

19. A
This is a time relationship. A turntable is an early type of stereo, MP3 player is a modern stereo. In the same way, a horse drawn carriage is an earlier type of car.

20. A
This is a type relationship. A cub is a young bear, in the same way a puppy is a young dog.

Section V – Science

1. C
Electric potential is a fundamental interaction between the magnetic field and the presence and motion of an electric charge. Electric potential is the capacity of an electric field to do work on an electric charge, typically measured in volts, while electromagnetism is a fundamental interaction between the magnetic field and the

presence and motion of an electric charge

2. D
An ohm (Ω) is a unit of electrical voltage is not true.
Note: An ohm is a unit of electrical resistance.

3. D
The property of a conductor that restricts its internal flow of electrons is **resistance**.

4. C
In physics, friction is the force that opposes the relative motion of two bodies in contact.

5. B
Kinetic energy is the energy of a body that results from motion while potential energy is the energy possessed by an object by virtue of its position or state, e.g., as in a compressed spring.

6. A
The four fundamental forces of nature are gravity, electromagnetic force, weak nuclear force, and strong nuclear force.
Note: Electromagnetic force is more commonly known as electricity.

7. A
Starting with the weakest, the fundamental forces of nature in order of strength are, Gravity, Weak nuclear force, Electromagnetic force, Strong nuclear force.
Note: Although gravitational force is the weakest of the four, it acts over great distances. Electromagnetic force is of order 1039 times stronger than gravity.[15]

8. A
The Strong Nuclear Force is an attractive force that binds protons and neutrons and maintains the structure of the nucleus, and the Weak Nuclear Force is responsible for the radioactive beta decay and other subatomic reactions.

Note: The Weak Nuclear Force is so named because it is only effective for short distances. Nevertheless, it is through the Weak Nuclear Force that the sun provides us with energy by allowing one element to change into another element.[15]

9. B
No detectable gain or loss occurs in chemical reactions.

Note: No detectable gain or loss in mass occurs in chemical reactions. However, the state of a substance may change in a chemical reaction. For example, substances involving in a chemical reaction can change from solid states to gaseous states but the total mass will not change.[9]

10. C
Convection is the transfer of heat from one place to another by the movement of fluids; thermal radiation is electromagnetic radiation emitted from all matter due to its possessing thermal energy.

Note: In physics, the term "fluid" means any substance that deforms under shear stress; it includes liquids, gases, plasmas, and some plastic solids. Sunlight is solar electromagnetic radiation generated by the hot plasma of the Sun, and this thermal radiation heats the Earth.[16]

11. D
In **Eukaryotic** cells, the cell cycle is the cycle of events involving cell division, including **mitosis**, **cytokinesis**, and **interphase**.

12. D
All of these statements are true.

13. C
DNA is a nucleic acid that carries the genetic information in the cell and is capable of self-replication.

14. A
The complementary bases found in DNA are **adenine** and **thymine** or **cytosine** and **guanine**.

15. B
A **nucleotide** is the basic structural unit of nucleic acids (DNA or RNA); their sequence determines individual hereditary characteristics.

16. B
Ribonucleic acid (RNA) is a **chain of nucleotides** that plays an important role in the creation of new **proteins**.

17. C
Mutations in DNA sequences usually occur spontaneously is false.

Note: Mutations result when the DNA polymerase makes a mistake, which happens about once every 100,000,000 bases. Actually, the number of mistakes that remain incorporated into the DNA is even lower than this because cells contain special DNA repair proteins that fix many of the mistakes in the DNA that are caused by mutagens. The repair proteins see which nucleotides are paired incorrectly, and then change the wrong base to the right one.[17]

18. A
Aerobic reactions occur in every cell and use **oxygen** to convert glucose to energy; **anaerobic** organisms such as many bacteria can release energy without the use of **oxygen**.

19. D
Tissues are a collection of similar cells that group together to perform a specialized function.

20. A
Epithelial tissue serves as membranes lining organs and helping to keep the body's organs separate, in place and protected; an example is the outer layer of the skin.

21. D
Tissue that adds support and structure to the body and frequently contains fibrous strands of collagen is **connective** tissue.

22. B
Muscle tissue is a specialized tissue that can contract and contains the specialized proteins actin and myosin that slide past one another and allow movement.

23. A
Nerve tissue contains two types of cells: neurons and glial cells and has the ability to generate and conduct electrical signals in the body.

24. D
An organ is a group of tissues that perform a specific function or group of functions.

25. B
Among animals, examples of **organs** are the heart, lungs, brain, eye, stomach, and bones; plant **organs** include the roots, stems, leaves, flowers, seeds and fruits.

26. C
Our bodies have **11** different **systems**, including **circulatory, digestive**, and **lymphatic**.

Note: Other systems include the endocrine, immune, muscular, nervous, reproductive, respiratory, skeletal, and urinary systems.

27. D
The Lymphatic system absorbs excess fluid, preventing tissues from swelling, defends the body against microorganisms and harmful foreign particles, and facilitates the absorption of fat.

28. A
The **vascular** system consists of **arteries, veins**, and **capillaries** that transport oxygen to and from all tissues.

29. D
Arteries carry oxygenated blood away from the heart, veins return oxygen-depleted

blood to the heart, and capillaries are thin-walled blood vessels in which gas/ nutrient/ waste exchange occurs.

Note: An easy way to remember the difference between an artery and a vein is that Arteries carry Away from the heart.

30. B
The small **intestine** is the primary organ of the digestive tract, and may be subdivided into three segments, the **duodenum**, the **jejunum**, and the **ileum**.

31. B
The **immune** system defends our bodies against infections and disease through three types of response systems: the **anatomic** response, the **inflammatory** response, and the **immune** response.

32. A
The **musculoskeletal** system is composed of all of the bones, cartilage, muscles, joints, tendons and ligaments in a person's body.

Note: Some people view the musculoskeletal system as two body systems that work very closely together.[18]

33. C
The **gastrointestinal** tract is a muscular tube lined by a special layer of cells, called **epithelium**; its primary purpose is to break food down into **nutrients**, which can be absorbed into the body to provide energy.

34. C
The **Law of the Conservation of Energy** states that, in a chemical change, **energy** can be neither **created** nor **destroyed**, but only changed from **one form to another**.

35. C
A **chemical change** is a process that transforms one set of chemical substances to another; the substances used are known as **reactants** and those formed are products.

36. B
Oxygen is the most abundant element in the Earth's crust and appears on the Atomic Table as the letter **'O'**.

37. D
Anabolism is the series of chemical reactions resulting in the **synthesis** of organic compounds, and **catabolism** is a series of chemical reactions that **break down** larger molecules.

38. D
A **catalyst** is a chemical involved in, but not changed by, a chemical reaction by which chemical bonds are **weakened** and reactions **accelerated**.

Note: Enzymes function as organic catalysts and allow many chemical reactions to occur within the homeostatic constraints of a living system. Enzymes can act rapidly, as in the case of carbonic anhydrase (enzymes typically end in the -ase suffix), which causes the chemicals to react 107 times faster than without the enzyme present.

39. A
The Law of Multiple Proportions states that when two elements combine with each other to form more than one compound, the weights of one element that combine with a fixed weight of the other are in a ratio of small whole numbers.

40. D
The Law of Definite Proportions states that every chemical compound contains fixed and constant proportions (by weight) of its constituent elements.
Note: Although many experimenters had long assumed the truth of the principle in general, the French chemist Joseph-Louis Proust first accumulated conclusive evidence for it in a series of researches on the composition of many substances, especially the oxides of iron (1797).[19]

41. C
The Pauli Exclusion Principle states that, in a given **molecule, no two electrons can** have **a different set of four quantum numbers**.
42. B
According to the tenets of Dalton's atomic theory, **All atoms of an element are alike in weight, and this weight is specific to the kind of atom.**

43. A
Atoms of **different elements** combine in **simple whole-number** ratios to form chemical **compounds**.

44. B
The following statement about the periodic table is true, **the way in which the elements are arranged allows predictions to made about their behavior.**

45. A
Ionization energy is the minimum quantity of energy required to remove an electron from an atom or ion in the gas phase.

46. D
An **atomic radius** is one-half the distance between nuclei of atoms of the same element, when the atoms are bound by a single covalent bond or are in a metallic crystal.

47. A & B are correct.
An anion is a negatively charged ion, and a cation is a positively charged ion. Anions are typically formed by nonmetals, and metals usually form cations.

48. C
The radius of atoms obtained from **covalent** bond lengths is called the **covalent** radius; the radius from interatomic distances in metallic crystals is called the **metallic** radius.

49. D
A **periodic trend** is a regular variation in element properties with **increasing** atomic number that is ultimately due to **regular** variations in atomic structure.

50. D
All of these statements are true.

Practice Test Questions Set 2

THE PRACTICE TEST PORTION PRESENTS QUESTIONS THAT ARE REPRESENTATIVE OF THE TYPE OF QUESTION YOU SHOULD EXPECT TO FIND ON THE DET. However, they are not intended to match exactly what is on the DET.

For the best results, take this Practice Test as if it were the real exam. Set aside time when you will not be disturbed, and a location that is quiet and free of distractions. Read the instructions carefully, read each question carefully, and answer to the best of your ability.

Use the bubble answer sheets provided. When you have completed the Practice Test, check your answer against the Answer Key and read the explanation provided.

NOTE: The Science, Anatomy and Physiology and English sections are optional. Check with your school for exam details.

Reading Comprehension Answer Sheet

1. (A) (B) (C) (D)	18. (A) (B) (C) (D)	35. (A) (B) (C) (D)
2. (A) (B) (C) (D)	19. (A) (B) (C) (D)	36. (A) (B) (C) (D)
3. (A) (B) (C) (D)	20. (A) (B) (C) (D)	37. (A) (B) (C) (D)
4. (A) (B) (C) (D)	21. (A) (B) (C) (D)	38. (A) (B) (C) (D)
5. (A) (B) (C) (D)	22. (A) (B) (C) (D)	39. (A) (B) (C) (D)
6. (A) (B) (C) (D)	23. (A) (B) (C) (D)	40. (A) (B) (C) (D)
7. (A) (B) (C) (D)	24. (A) (B) (C) (D)	41. (A) (B) (C) (D)
8. (A) (B) (C) (D)	25. (A) (B) (C) (D)	42. (A) (B) (C) (D)
9. (A) (B) (C) (D)	26. (A) (B) (C) (D)	43. (A) (B) (C) (D)
10. (A) (B) (C) (D)	27. (A) (B) (C) (D)	44. (A) (B) (C) (D)
11. (A) (B) (C) (D)	28. (A) (B) (C) (D)	45. (A) (B) (C) (D)
12. (A) (B) (C) (D)	29. (A) (B) (C) (D)	46. (A) (B) (C) (D)
13. (A) (B) (C) (D)	30. (A) (B) (C) (D)	47. (A) (B) (C) (D)
14. (A) (B) (C) (D)	31. (A) (B) (C) (D)	48. (A) (B) (C) (D)
15. (A) (B) (C) (D)	32. (A) (B) (C) (D)	49. (A) (B) (C) (D)
16. (A) (B) (C) (D)	33. (A) (B) (C) (D)	50. (A) (B) (C) (D)
17. (A) (B) (C) (D)	34. (A) (B) (C) (D)	

Math Answer Sheet

1. (A) (B) (C) (D)
2. (A) (B) (C) (D)
3. (A) (B) (C) (D)
4. (A) (B) (C) (D)
5. (A) (B) (C) (D)
6. (A) (B) (C) (D)
7. (A) (B) (C) (D)
8. (A) (B) (C) (D)
9. (A) (B) (C) (D)
10. (A) (B) (C) (D)
11. (A) (B) (C) (D)
12. (A) (B) (C) (D)
13. (A) (B) (C) (D)
14. (A) (B) (C) (D)
15. (A) (B) (C) (D)
16. (A) (B) (C) (D)
17. (A) (B) (C) (D)
18. (A) (B) (C) (D)
19. (A) (B) (C) (D)
20. (A) (B) (C) (D)
21. (A) (B) (C) (D)
22. (A) (B) (C) (D)
23. (A) (B) (C) (D)
24. (A) (B) (C) (D)
25. (A) (B) (C) (D)
26. (A) (B) (C) (D)
27. (A) (B) (C) (D)
28. (A) (B) (C) (D)
29. (A) (B) (C) (D)
30. (A) (B) (C) (D)
31. (A) (B) (C) (D)
32. (A) (B) (C) (D)
33. (A) (B) (C) (D)
34. (A) (B) (C) (D)
35. (A) (B) (C) (D)
36. (A) (B) (C) (D)
37. (A) (B) (C) (D)
38. (A) (B) (C) (D)
39. (A) (B) (C) (D)
40. (A) (B) (C) (D)
41. (A) (B) (C) (D)
42. (A) (B) (C) (D)
43. (A) (B) (C) (D)
44. (A) (B) (C) (D)
45. (A) (B) (C) (D)
46. (A) (B) (C) (D)
47. (A) (B) (C) (D)
48. (A) (B) (C) (D)
49. (A) (B) (C) (D)
50. (A) (B) (C) (D)

English Grammar Answer Sheet

1. (A) (B) (C) (D)
2. (A) (B) (C) (D)
3. (A) (B) (C) (D)
4. (A) (B) (C) (D)
5. (A) (B) (C) (D)
6. (A) (B) (C) (D)
7. (A) (B) (C) (D)
8. (A) (B) (C) (D)
9. (A) (B) (C) (D)
10. (A) (B) (C) (D)
11. (A) (B) (C) (D)
12. (A) (B) (C) (D)
13. (A) (B) (C) (D)
14. (A) (B) (C) (D)
15. (A) (B) (C) (D)
16. (A) (B) (C) (D)
17. (A) (B) (C) (D)
18. (A) (B) (C) (D)
19. (A) (B) (C) (D)
20. (A) (B) (C) (D)
21. (A) (B) (C) (D)
22. (A) (B) (C) (D)
23. (A) (B) (C) (D)
24. (A) (B) (C) (D)
25. (A) (B) (C) (D)
26. (A) (B) (C) (D)
27. (A) (B) (C) (D)
28. (A) (B) (C) (D)
29. (A) (B) (C) (D)
30. (A) (B) (C) (D)
31. (A) (B) (C) (D)
32. (A) (B) (C) (D)
33. (A) (B) (C) (D)
34. (A) (B) (C) (D)
35. (A) (B) (C) (D)
36. (A) (B) (C) (D)
37. (A) (B) (C) (D)
38. (A) (B) (C) (D)
39. (A) (B) (C) (D)
40. (A) (B) (C) (D)
41. (A) (B) (C) (D)
42. (A) (B) (C) (D)
43. (A) (B) (C) (D)
44. (A) (B) (C) (D)
45. (A) (B) (C) (D)
46. (A) (B) (C) (D)
47. (A) (B) (C) (D)
48. (A) (B) (C) (D)
49. (A) (B) (C) (D)
50. (A) (B) (C) (D)

Critical Thinking Answer Sheet

1.	A	B	C	D	**11.**	A	B	C	D
2.	A	B	C	D	**12.**	A	B	C	D
3.	A	B	C	D	**13.**	A	B	C	D
4.	A	B	C	D	**14.**	A	B	C	D
5.	A	B	C	D	**15.**	A	B	C	D
6.	A	B	C	D	**16.**	A	B	C	D
7.	A	B	C	D	**17.**	A	B	C	D
8.	A	B	C	D	**18.**	A	B	C	D
9.	A	B	C	D	**19.**	A	B	C	D
10.	A	B	C	D	**20.**	A	B	C	D

Answer Sheet Section V - Basic Science

1. (A) (B) (C) (D)	18. (A) (B) (C) (D)	35. (A) (B) (C) (D)
2. (A) (B) (C) (D)	19. (A) (B) (C) (D)	36. (A) (B) (C) (D)
3. (A) (B) (C) (D)	20. (A) (B) (C) (D)	37. (A) (B) (C) (D)
4. (A) (B) (C) (D)	21. (A) (B) (C) (D)	38. (A) (B) (C) (D)
5. (A) (B) (C) (D)	22. (A) (B) (C) (D)	39. (A) (B) (C) (D)
6. (A) (B) (C) (D)	23. (A) (B) (C) (D)	40. (A) (B) (C) (D)
7. (A) (B) (C) (D)	24. (A) (B) (C) (D)	41. (A) (B) (C) (D)
8. (A) (B) (C) (D)	25. (A) (B) (C) (D)	42. (A) (B) (C) (D)
9. (A) (B) (C) (D)	26. (A) (B) (C) (D)	43. (A) (B) (C) (D)
10. (A) (B) (C) (D)	27. (A) (B) (C) (D)	44. (A) (B) (C) (D)
11. (A) (B) (C) (D)	28. (A) (B) (C) (D)	45. (A) (B) (C) (D)
12. (A) (B) (C) (D)	29. (A) (B) (C) (D)	46. (A) (B) (C) (D)
13. (A) (B) (C) (D)	30. (A) (B) (C) (D)	47. (A) (B) (C) (D)
14. (A) (B) (C) (D)	31. (A) (B) (C) (D)	48. (A) (B) (C) (D)
15. (A) (B) (C) (D)	32. (A) (B) (C) (D)	49. (A) (B) (C) (D)
16. (A) (B) (C) (D)	33. (A) (B) (C) (D)	50. (A) (B) (C) (D)
17. (A) (B) (C) (D)	34. (A) (B) (C) (D)	

Section I - Reading Comprehension

Questions 1-4 refer to the following passage.

Passage 1 - The Respiratory System

The respiratory system's function is to allow oxygen exchange through all parts of the body. The anatomy or structure of the exchange system, and the uses of the exchanged gases, varies depending on the organism. In humans and other mammals, for example, the anatomical features of the respiratory system include airways, lungs, and the respiratory muscles. Molecules of oxygen and carbon dioxide are passively exchanged, by diffusion, between the gaseous external environment and the blood. This exchange process occurs in the alveolar region of the lungs.

Other animals, such as insects, have respiratory systems with very simple anatomical features, and in amphibians even the skin plays a vital role in gas exchange. Plants also have respiratory systems but the direction of gas exchange can be opposite to that of animals.

The respiratory system can also be divided into physiological, or functional, zones. These include the conducting zone (the region for gas transport from the outside atmosphere to just above the alveoli), the transitional zone, and the respiratory zone (the alveolar region where gas exchange occurs). [19]

1. What can we infer from the first paragraph in this passage?

a. Human and mammal respiratory systems are the same.
b. The lungs are an important part of the respiratory system.
c. The respiratory system varies in different mammals.
d. Oxygen and carbon dioxide are passive exchanged by the respiratory system.

2. What is the process by which molecules of oxygen and carbon dioxide are passively exchanged?

a. Transfusion
b. Affusion
c. Diffusion
d. Respiratory confusion

3. What organ plays an important role in gas exchange in amphibians?

a. The skin
b. The lungs
c. The gills
d. The mouth

4. What are the three physiological zones of the respiratory system?

a. Conducting, transitional, respiratory zones
b. Redacting, transitional, circulatory zones
c. Conducting, circulatory, inhibiting zones
d. Transitional, inhibiting, conducting zones

Questions 5 - 8 refer to the following passage.

The Civil War

The Civil War began on April 12, 1861. The first shots of the Civil War were fired in Fort Sumter, South Carolina. Note that even though more American lives were lost in the Civil War than in any other war, not one person died on that first day. The war began because eleven Southern states seceded from the Union and tried to start their own government, The Confederate States of America.

Why did the states secede? The issue of slavery was a primary cause of the Civil War. The eleven southern states relied heavily on their slaves to foster their farming and plantation lifestyles. The northern states, many of whom had already abolished slavery, did not feel that the southern states should have slaves. The north wanted to free all the slaves and President Lincoln's goal was to both end slavery and preserve the Union. He had Congress declare war on the Confederacy on April 14, 1862. For four long, blood soaked years, the North and South fought.

From 1861 to mid 1863, it seemed as if the South would win this war. However, on July 1, 1863, an epic three day battle was waged on a field in Gettysburg, Pennsylvania. Gettysburg is remembered for being the bloodiest battle in American history. At the end of the three days, the North turned the tide of the war in their favor. The North then went on to dominate the South for the remainder of the war. Most well remembered might be General Sherman's "March to The Sea," where he famously led the Union Army through Georgia and the Carolinas, burning and destroying everything in their path.

In 1865, the Union army invaded and captured the Confederate capital of Richmond Virginia. Robert E. Lee, leader of the Confederacy surrendered to General Ulysses S. Grant, leader of the Union forces, on April 9, 1865. The Civil War was over, and the Union was preserved.

5. What does the word secede most nearly mean?

a. To break away from
b. To accomplish
c. To join
d. To lose

6. Which of the following statements summarizes a FACT from the passage?

a. Congress declared war and then the Battle of Fort Sumter began.
b. Congress declared war after shots were fired at Fort Sumter.
c. President Lincoln was pro slavery
d. President Lincoln was at Fort Sumter with Congress

7. Which event finally led the Confederacy to surrender?

a. The battle of Gettysburg
b. The battle of Bull Run
c. The invasion of the confederate capital of Richmond
d. Sherman's March to the Sea

8. The word abolish as used in this passage most nearly means?

a. To ban
b. To polish
c. To support
d. To destroy

Questions 9 – 11 refer to the following passage.

Passage 2 – Mythology

The main characters in myths are usually gods or supernatural heroes. As sacred stories, rulers and priests have traditionally endorsed their myths and as a result, myths have a close link with religion and politics. In the society where a myth originates, the natives believe the myth is a true account of the remote past. In fact, many societies have two categories of traditional narrative—(1) "true stories," or myths, and (2) "false stories," or fables.

Myths generally take place during a primordial age, when the world was still young, prior to achieving its current form. These stories explain how the world gained its current form and why the culture developed its customs, institutions, and taboos. Closely related to myth are legend and folktale. Myths, legends, and folktales are different types of traditional stories. Unlike myths, folktales can take place at any time and any place, and the natives do not usually consider them true or sacred. Legends, on the other hand, are similar to myths in that many people have traditionally considered them true. Legends take place in a more recent time, when the world was much as it is today. In addition, legends generally feature humans as their main characters, whereas myths have super-human characters. [20]

9. We can infer from this passage that

a. Folktales took place in a time far past, before civilization covered the earth.

b. Humankind uses myth to explain how the world was created.

c. Myths revolve around gods or supernatural beings; the local community usually accepts these stories as not true.

d. The only difference between a myth and a legend is the time setting of the story.

10. The main purpose of this passage is

a. To distinguish between many types of traditional stories, and explain the background of some traditional story categories.

b. To determine whether myths and legends might be true accounts of history.

c. To show the importance of folktales how these traditional stories made life more bearable in harder times.

d. None of the Above.

11. How are folktales different from myths?

a. Folktales and myth are the same.

b. Folktales are not true and generally not sacred and take place anytime.

c. Myths are not true and generally not sacred and take place anytime.

d. Folktales explained the formation of the world and myths do not.

Questions 12 refers to the following table of contents.

Getting Started

12. Based on the partial table of contents above, what is this book about?

a. How to answer multiple choice questions

b. Different types of multiple choice questions

c. How to write a test

d. None of the above

Questions 13 - 16 refer to the following passage.

Passage 3 – Myths, Legend and Folklore

Cultural historians draw a distinction between myth, legend and folktale simply as a way to group traditional stories. However, in many cultures, drawing a sharp line between myths and legends is not that simple. Instead of dividing their traditional stories into myths, legends, and folktales, some cultures divide them into two categories. The first category roughly corresponds with folktales, and the second is one that combines myths and legends. Similarly, we cannot always separate myths from folktales. One society might consider a story true, making it a myth. Another society may believe the story is fiction, which makes it a folktale. In fact, when a myth loses its status as part of a religious system, it often takes on traits more typical of folktales, with its formerly divine characters now appearing as human heroes, giants, or fairies. Myth, legend, and folktale are only a few of the categories of traditional stories. Other categories include anecdotes and some kinds of jokes. Traditional stories, in turn, are only one category within the larger category of folklore, which also includes items such as gestures, costumes, and music. [20]

13. The main idea of this passage is that

a. Myths, fables, and folktales are not the same thing, and each describes a specific type of story.

b. Traditional stories can be categorized in different ways by different people.

c. Cultures use myths for religious purposes, and when this is no longer true, the people forget and discard these myths.

d. Myths can never become folk tales, because one is true, and the other is false.

14. The terms myth and legend are

a. Categories that are synonymous with true and false.

b. Categories that group traditional stories according to certain characteristics.

c. Interchangeable, because both terms mean a story that is passed down from generation to generation.

d. Meant to distinguish between a story that involves a hero and a cultural message and a story meant only to entertain.

15. Traditional story categories not only include myths and legends, but

a. Can also include gestures, since some cultures passed these down before the written and spoken word.

b. In addition, folklore refers to stories involving fables and fairy tales.

c. These story categories can also include folk music and traditional dress.

d. Traditional stories themselves are a part of the larger category of folklore, which may also include costumes, gestures, and music.

16. This passage shows that

a. There is a distinct difference between a myth and a legend, although, both are folktales.

b. Myths are folktales, but folktales are not myths.

c. Myths, legends, and folktales play an important part in tradition and the past, and are a rich and colorful part of history.

d. Most cultures consider myths to be true.

Questions 17 - 20 refer to the following passage.

A Day That Will Live in Infamy! Attack on Pearl Harbor

In 1941, the world was at war. The United States was trying very hard to keep itself out of the conflict. In Europe, the countries of Germany and Italy had formed an alliance to expand their land and territory. Germany had already taken over Poland, Denmark, and parts of France. They were heading next toward England and due to all the fighting in Europe, there were battles taking place as far south as North Africa, where the German and Italian armies were fighting the British.

This got even worse when the Asian nation of Japan formed an alliance with Germany and Italy. Together, the three countries called themselves, the AXIS. Now, the war was in the Pacific as well as in Europe and Northern Africa. Many Americans felt that perhaps now was the time for the United States to join with its ally, Great Britain and stop the Axis from taking over more regions of the world.

In 1941, Franklin Roosevelt was President of the United States. His fear at the time was that Japan would try to take over many countries in Asia. He did not want to see that happen, so he moved some of the United States warships that had been stationed in San Diego, to the military base at Pearl Harbor, in Honolulu, Hawaii.

Japan quietly plotted their attack. They waited until the early hours of the morning on Sunday, December 7, 1941. Then, 350 Japanese war plans began to drop bombs on the U.S. ships at Pearl Harbor.

The first bombs fell at 7:48 am and a mere 90 minutes later, the attack was over. Pearl

Harbor was decimated. 8 battleships were damaged. Eleven ships were sunk and 300 U.S. planes were destroyed. Most devastating was the loss of life 2,400 U.S. military members was killed in the attack and 1, 282 were injured.

President Roosevelt addressed the country via the radio and said "Today is a day that will live in infamy." He asked Congress to declare war on Japan. War was declared on Japan on December 8th and on Germany and Italy on December 11th. The United States had entered World War Two.

17. After reading the passage, what can we infer the word infamy means?

a. Famous
b. Remembered in a good way
c. Remembered in a bad way
d. Easily forgotten

18. What three countries formed the Axis?

a. Italy, England, Germany
b. United States, England, Italy
c. Germany, Japan, Italy
d. Germany, Japan, United States

19. What do you think was President Roosevelt's reason for moving warships to Pearl Harbor?

a. He feared Japan would bomb San Diego
b. He knew Japan was going to attack Pearl Harbor
c. He was planning to attack Japan
d. He wanted to try and protect Asian countries from Japanese takeover

20. Why do you think Japan chose a Sunday morning at 7:48am for their attack?

a. They knew the military slept late
b. There is a law against bombing countries on a Sunday
c. They wanted the attack to catch people by surprise
d. That was the only free time they had to attack.

Questions 21 - 24 refer to the following passage.

The Winged Victory of Samothrace: the Statue of the Gods

Students who read about the "Winged Victory of Samothrace" probably won't be able to picture what this statue looks like. However, almost anyone who knows a little about statues will recognize it when they see it: it is the statue of a winged woman who does not have arms or a head. Even the most famous pieces of art may be recognized by sight but not by name.

This iconic statue is of the Greek goddess Nike, who represented victory and was called Victoria by the Romans. The statue is sometimes called the "Nike of Samothrace." She was often displayed in Greek art as driving a chariot, and her speed or efficiency with the chariot may be what her wings symbolize. It is said that the statue was created around 200 BCE to celebrate a battle that was won at sea. Archaeologists and art historians believe the statue may have originally been part of a temple or other building, even one of the most important temples, Megaloi Theoi, just as many statues were used during that time.

"Winged Victory" does indeed appear to have had arms and a head when it was originally created, and it is unclear why they were removed or lost. Indeed, they have never been discovered, even with all the excavation that has taken place. Many speculate that one of her arms was raised and put to her mouth, as though she was shouting or calling out, which is consistent with the idea of her as a war figure. If the missing pieces were ever to be found, they might give Greek and art historians more of an idea of what Nike represented or how the statue was used.

Learning about pieces of art through details like these can help students remember time frames or locations, as well as learn about the people who occupied them.

21. The author's title says the statue is "of the Gods" because

a. the statue is very beautiful and even a god would find it beautiful

b. the statue is of a Greek goddess, and gods were of primary importance to the Greek

c. Nike lead the gods into war

d. the statues were used at the temple of the gods and so it belonged to them

22. The third paragraph states that

a. the statue is related to war and was probably broken apart by foreign soldiers

b. the arms and head of the statue cannot be found because all the excavation has taken place

c. speculations have been made about what the entire statue looked like and what it symbolized

d. the statue has no arms or head because the sculptor lost them

23. The author's main purpose in writing this passage is to

a. demonstrate that art and culture are related and one can teach us about the other

b. persuade readers to become archeologists and find the missing pieces of the statue

c. teach readers about the Greek goddess Nike

d. to teach readers the name of a statue they probably recognize

24. The author specifies the indirect audience as "students" because

a. it is probably a student who is taking this test

b. most young people don't know much about art yet and most young people are students

c. students read more than people who are not students

d. the passage is based on a discussion of what we can learn about culture from art

Questions 25 - 27 refer to the following passage.

Lowest Price Guarantee

Get it for less. Guaranteed!

ABC Electric will beat any advertised price by 10% of the difference.

1) If you find a lower advertised price, we will beat it by 10% of the difference.

2) If you find a lower advertised price within 30 days* of your purchase we will beat it by 10% of the difference.

3) If our own price is reduced within 30 days* of your purchase, bring in your receipt and we will refund the difference.

*14 days for computers, monitors, printers, laptops, tablets, cellular & wireless devices, home security products, projectors, camcorders, digital cameras, radar detectors, portable DVD players, DJ and pro-audio equipment, and air conditioners.

25. I bought a radar detector 15 days ago and saw an ad for the same model only cheaper. Can I get 10% of the difference refunded?

a. Yes. Since it is less than 30 days, you can get 10% of the difference refunded.

b. No. Since it is more than 14 days, you cannot get 10% of the difference refunded.

c. It depends on the cashier.

d. Yes. You can get the difference refunded.

26. I bought a flat-screen TV for $500 10 days ago and found an advertisement for the same TV, at another store, on sale for $400. How much will ABC refund under this guarantee?

a. $100
b. $110
c. $10
d. $400

27. What is the purpose of this passage?

a. To inform
b. To educate
c. To persuade
d. To entertain

Questions 28 - 31 refer to the following passage.

Ways Characters Communicate in Theater

Playwrights give their characters voices in a way that gives depth and added meaning to what happens on stage during their play. There are different types of speech in scripts that allow characters to talk with themselves, with other characters, and even with the audience.

It is very unique to theater that characters may talk "to themselves." When characters do this, the speech they give is called a soliloquy. Soliloquies are usually poetic, introspective, moving, and can tell audience members about the feelings, motivations, or suspicions of an individual character without that character having to reveal them to other characters on stage. "To be or not to be" is a famous soliloquy given by Hamlet as he considers difficult but important themes, such as life and death.

The most common type of communication in plays is when one character is speaking to another or a group of other characters. This is generally called dialogue, but can also be called monologue if one character speaks without being interrupted for a long time. It is not necessarily the most important type of communication, but it is the most common because the plot of the play cannot really progress without it.
Lastly, and most unique to theater (although it has been used somewhat in film) is when a character speaks directly to the audience. This is called an aside, and scripts usually specifically direct actors to do this. Asides are usually comical, an inside joke between the character and the audience, and very short. The actor will usually face the audience when delivering them, even if it's for a moment, so the audience can recognize

this move as an aside.

All three of these types of communication are important to the art of theater, and have been perfected by famous playwrights like Shakespeare. Understanding these types of communication can help an audience member grasp what is artful about the script and action of a play.

28. According to the passage, characters in plays communicate to

a. move the plot forward
b. show the private thoughts and feelings of one character
c. make the audience laugh
d. add beauty and artistry to the play

29. When Hamlet delivers "To be or not to be," he can most likely be described as

a. solitary
b. thoughtful
c. dramatic
d. hopeless

30. The author uses parentheses to punctuate "although it has been used somewhat in film"

a. to show that films are less important
b. instead of using commas so that the sentence is not interrupted
c. because parenthesis help separate details that are not as important
d. to show that films are not as artistic

31. It can be understood that by the phrase "give their characters voices," the author means that

a. playwrights are generous
b. playwrights are changing the sound or meaning of characters' voices to fit what they had in mind
c. dialogue is important in creating characters
d. playwrights may be the parent of one of their actors and literally give them their voice

Questions 32 - 35 refer to the following passage.

The Circulatory System

The circulatory system is an organ system that passes nutrients (such as amino acids and electrolytes), gases, hormones, and blood cells to and from cells in the body to help fight diseases and help stabilize body temperature and pH levels.

The circulatory system may be seen strictly as a blood distribution network, but some consider the circulatory system as composed of the cardiovascular system, which distributes blood, and the lymphatic system, which distributes lymph. While humans, as well as other vertebrates, have a closed cardiovascular system (meaning that the blood never leaves the network of arteries, veins and capillaries), some invertebrate groups have an open cardiovascular system. The most primitive animal phyla lack circulatory systems. The lymphatic system, on the other hand, is an open system.

Two types of fluids move through the circulatory system: blood and lymph. The blood, heart, and blood vessels form the cardiovascular system. The lymph, the lymph nodes, and lymph vessels form the lymphatic system. The cardiovascular system and the lymphatic system collectively make up the circulatory system.

The main components of the human cardiovascular system are the heart and the blood vessels. It includes: the pulmonary circulation, a "loop" through the lungs where blood is oxygenated; and the systemic circulation, a "loop" through the rest of the body to provide oxygenated blood. An average adult contains five to six quarts (roughly 4.7 to 5.7 liters) of blood, which consists of plasma, red blood cells, white blood cells, and platelets. Also, the digestive system works with the circulatory system to provide the nutrients the system needs to keep the heart pumping. [21]

32. What can we infer from the first paragraph?

a. An important purpose of the circulatory system is that of fighting diseases.

b. The most important function of the circulatory system is to give the person energy.

c. The least important function of the circulatory system is that of growing skin cells.

d. The entire purpose of the circulatory system is not known.

33. Do humans have an open or closed circulatory system?

a. Open

b. Closed

c. Usually open, though sometimes closed

d. Usually closed, though sometimes open

34. Besides blood, what two components form the cardiovascular system?

a. The heart and the lungs
b. The lungs and the veins
c. The heart and the blood vessels
d. The blood vessels and the nerves

35. Which system, along with the circulatory system, helps provide nutrients to keep the human heart pumping?

a. The skeletal system
b. The digestive system
c. The immune system
d. The nervous system

Questions 38 - 41 refer to the following passage.

Passage 8 - Blood

Blood is a specialized bodily fluid that delivers nutrients and oxygen to the body's cells and transports waste products away.

In vertebrates, blood consists of blood cells suspended in a liquid called blood plasma. Plasma, which comprises 55% of blood fluid, is mostly water (90% by volume), and contains dissolved proteins, glucose, mineral ions, hormones, carbon dioxide, platelets and the blood cells themselves.

Blood cells are mainly red blood cells (also called RBCs or erythrocytes) and white blood cells, including leukocytes and platelets. Red blood cells are the most abundant cells, and contain an iron-containing protein called hemoglobin that transports oxygen through the body.

The pumping action of the heart circulates blood around the body through blood vessels. In animals with lungs, arterial blood carries oxygen from inhaled air to the tissues of the body, and venous blood carries carbon dioxide, a waste product of metabolism produced by cells, from the tissues to the lungs to be exhaled. [22]

36. What can we infer from the first paragraph in this passage?

a. Blood is responsible for transporting oxygen to the cells.
b. Blood is only red when it reaches the outside of the body.
c. Each person has about six pints of blood.
d. Blood's true function was only learned in the last century.

37. What liquid are blood cells suspended?

a. Plasma
b. Water
c. Liquid nitrogen
d. A mixture consisting largely of human milk

38. Which of these is not contained in blood plasma?

a. Hormones
b. Mineral ions
c. Calcium
d. Glucose

39. Which body part exhales carbon dioxide after venous blood has carried it from body tissues?

a. The lungs
b. The skin cells
c. The bowels
d. The sweat glands

Question 40 refers to the following passage.

The Human Skeleton

The human skeleton consists of both fused and individual bones supported and supplemented by ligaments, tendons, muscles and cartilage. It serves as a scaffold which supports organs, anchors muscles, and protects organs such as the brain, lungs and heart. The biggest bone in the body is the femur in the upper leg, and the smallest is the stapes bone in the middle ear. In an adult, the skeleton comprises around 14% of the total body weight, and half of this weight is water.

Fused bones include the pelvis and the cranium. Not all bones are interconnected directly: There are three bones in each middle ear called the ossicles that articulate only with each other. The thyroid bone, which is located in the neck, and serves as the point of attachment for the tongue, does not articulate with any other bones in the body, being supported by muscles and ligaments.

There are 206 bones in the adult human skeleton, which varies between individuals and with age - newborn babies have over 270 bones, some of which fuse together. These bones are organized into a longitudinal axis, the axial skeleton, to which the appendicular skeleton is attached. [23]

40. What is the main idea of this passage?

a. The human skeleton is an important and complicated system of the body.

b. There are 206 bones in the typical human body.

c. In a child, the skeleton represents 14% of the body weight.

d. Bones become more fragile as we age.

Section II – Math

1. 8327 – 1278 =

a. 7149

b. 7209

c. 6059

d. 7049

2. 294 X 21 =

a. 6017

b. 6174

c. 6728

d. 5679

3. 1278 + 4920 =

a. 6298

b. 6108

c. 6198

d. 6098

4. 285 * 12 =

a. 3420

b. 3402

c. 3024

d. 2322

5. 4120 – 3216 =

a. 903

b. 804

c. 904

d. 1904

6. 2417 + 1004 =

a. 3401

b. 4321

c. 3402

d. 3421

7. 1440 ÷ 12 =

a. 122

b. 120

c. 110

d. 132

8. 2713 – 1308 =

a. 1450

b. 1445

c. 1405

d. 1455

9. It is known that $x^2+4x=5$. Then x can be

a. 0

b. -5

c. 1

d. Either (b) or (c)

10. (a+b)2 = 4ab. What is necessarily correct?

a. $a > b$
b. $a < b$
c. $a = b$
d. None of the Above

11. The sum of the digits of a 2-digit number is 12. If we switch the digits, the number we get will be greater than the initial one by 36. Find the initial number.

a. 39
b. 48
c. 57
d. 75

12. Two friends traveled to a nearby city. On the second day they travelled 75 miles more than the first day, and in the third day, they travelled a third of the distance covered in the second day. How many miles did they cover in the first day, if the total travelled was 170 miles?

a. 30 miles
b. 35 miles
c. 105 miles
d. 135 miles

13. Kate's father is 32 years older than Kate is. In 5 years, he will be five times older. How old is Kate?

a. 2
b. 3
c. 5
d. 6

14. If Lynn can type a page in p minutes, what portion of the page can she do in 5 minutes?

a. $5/p$
b. $p - 5$
c. $p + 5$
d. $p/5$

15. If Sally can paint a house in 4 hours, and John can paint the same house in 6 hours, how long will it take for both of them to paint the house together?

a. 2 hours and 24 minutes
b. 3 hours and 12 minutes
c. 3 hours and 44 minutes
d. 4 hours and 10 minutes

16. Employees of a discount appliance store receive an additional 20% off the lowest price on any item. If an employee purchases a dishwasher during a 15% off sale, how much will he pay if the dishwasher originally cost $450?

a. $280.90
b. $287
c. $292.50
d. $306

17. The sale price of a car is $12,590, which is 20% off the original price. What is the original price?

a. $14,310.40
b. $14,990.90
c. $15,108.00
d. $15,737.50

18. A goat eats 214 kg. of hay in 60 days, while a cow eats the same amount in 15 days. How long will it take them to eat this hay together?

a. 37.5
b. 75
c. 12
d. 15

19. Express 25% as a fraction.

a. 1/4
b. 7/40
c. 6/25
d. 8/28

20. Express 125% as a decimal.

a. .125
b. 12.5
c. 1.25
d. 125

21. Solve for x: 30 is 40% of x

a. 60
b. 90
c. 85
d. 75

22. 12 ½% of x is equal to 50. Solve for x.

a. 300
b. 400
c. 450
d. 350

23. Express 24/56 as a reduced common fraction.

a. 4/9
b. 4/11
c. 3/7
d. 3/8

24. Express 87% as a decimal.

a. .087
b. 8.7
c. .87
d. 87

25. 60 is 75% of x. Solve for x.

a. 80
b. 90
c. 75
d. 70

26. 60% of x is 12. Solve for x.

a. 18
b. 15
c. 25
d. 20

27. Express 71/1000 as a decimal.

a. .71
b. .0071
c. .071
d. 7.1

28. 4.7 + .9 + .01 =

a. 5.5
b. 6.51
c. 5.61
d. 5.7

29. .33 × .59 =

a. .1947
b. 1.947
c. .0197
d. .1817

30. .84 ÷ .7 =

a. .12
b. 12
c. .012
d. 1.2

31. What number is in the ten thousandths place in 1.7389?

a. 1
b. 8
c. 9
d. 3

32. .87 - .48 =

a. .39
b. .49
c. .41
d. .37

33. The physician ordered 100 mg Ibuprofen/kg of body weight; on hand is 230 mg/tablet. The child weighs 50 lb. How many tablets will you give?

a. 10 tablets
b. 5 tablets
c. 1 tablet
d. 12 tablets

34. The physician ordered 1,000 units of heparin; 5,000 U/mL is on hand. How many milliliters will you give?

a. 0.002 ml
b. 0.2 ml
c. 0.02 ml
d. 2 ml

35. Simplify 4^3

a. 20
b. 32
c. 64
d. 108

36. The physician ordered 5 mL of Capacitate; 15 mL/tsp is on hand. How many teaspoons will you give?

a. 0.05 tsp
b. 0.03 tsp
c. 0.5 tsp
d. 0.3 tsp

37. The physician orders 70 mg morphine sulphate; 1 g/mL is on hand. How many mL will you give?

a. 0.05 ml
b. 0.07 ml
c. 0.04 ml
d. 0.007 ml

38. The physician ordered 200 mg amoxicillin. The pharmacy stocks amoxicillin 400 mg per tsp. How many teaspoons will you give?

a. 0.55 tsp
b. 0.25 tsp
c. 0.5 tsp
d. 0.05 tsp

39. The physician ordered 600 mg ibuprofen; the office stocks 200 mg per tablet. How many tablets will you give?

a. 3.5 tablets
b. 2 tablets
c. 5 tablets
d. 3 tablets

40. The manager of a weaving factory estimates that if 10 machines run on 100% efficiency for 8 hours, they will produce 1450 meters of cloth. However, due to some technical problems, 4 machines run of 95% efficiency and the remaining 6 at 90% efficiency. How many meters of cloth can these machines will produce in 8 hours?

a. 1334 meters
b. 1310 meters
c. 1300 meters
d. 1285 meters

41. Convert 60 feet to inches.

a. 700 inches
b. 600 inches
c. 720 inches
d. 1,800 inches

42. Convert 25 centimeters to millimeters.

a. 250 millimeters
b. 7.5 millimeters
c. 5 millimeters
d. 2.5 millimeters

43. Convert 100 millimeters to centimeters.

a. 10 centimeters
b. 1,000 centimeters
c. 1100 centimeters
d. 50 centimeters

44. Convert 3 gallons to quarts.

a. 15 quarts
b. 6 quarts
c. 12 quarts
d. 32 quarts

45. 2000 mm. =

a. 2 m
b. 200 m
c. 0.002 m
d. 0.02 m

46. 0.05 ml. =

a. 50 liters
b. 0.00005 liters
c. 5 liters
d. 0.0005 liters

47. 30 mg is the same mass as:

a. 0.0003 kg.
b. 0.03 grams
c. 300 decigrams
d. 0.3 grams

48. 0.101 mm. =

a. .0101 cm
b. 1.01 cm
c. 0.00101 cm
d. 10.10 cm

49. How much water can be stored in a cylindrical container 5 meters in diameter and 12 meters high?

a. $223.65m^3$
b. $235.65m^3$
c. $240.65m^3$
d. $252.65m^3$

50. Smith and Simon are playing a card game. Smith will win if a card drawn from a deck of 52 is either 7 or a diamond, and Simon will win if the drawn card is an even number. Which statement is more likely to be correct?

a. Smith will win more games.
b. Simon will win more games.
c. They have same winning probability.
d. A decision cannot be made from the provided data.

Section III – English Grammar

1. Elaine promised to bring the camera _______________ at the mall yesterday.

a. by me
b. with me
c. at me
d. to me

2. Last night, he _____________ the sleeping bag down beside my mattress.

a. lay
b. laid
c. lain
d. has laid

3. I would have bought the shirt for you if _________________.

a. I had known you liked it.
b. I have known you liked it.
c. I would know you liked it.
d. I know you liked it.

4. Many believers still hope _________________ proof of the existence of ghosts.

a. two find
b. to find
c. to found
d. to have been found

Fill in the blank.

5. All of the people at the school, including the teachers and ______________ were glad when summer break came.

a. students:
b. students,
c. students;
d. students

6. To _____________, Anne was on time for her math class.

a. everybody's surprise
b. every body's surprise
c. everybodys surprise
d. everybodys' surprise

7. If he ______________ the textbook like he was supposed to, he would have known what was on the test.

a. will have read
b. shouldn't have read
c. would have read
d. had read

8. Following the tornado, telephone poles _____________ all over the street.

a. laid
b. lied
c. were lying
d. were laying

9. In Edgar Allen Poe's ____________________ Edgar Allen Poe describes a man with a guilty conscience.

a. short story, "The Tell-Tale Heart,"
b. short story The Tell-Tale Heart,
c. short story, The Tell-Tale Heart
d. short story. "the Tell-Tale Heart,"

10. Billboards are considered an important part of advertising for big business, ______________ by their critics.

a. but, an eyesore;
b. but, " an eyesore,"
c. but an eyesore
d. but-an eyesore-

11. I can never remember how to use those two common words, "sell," meaning to trade a product for money, or _________________ meaning an event where products are traded for less money than usual.

a. sale-
b. "sale,"
c. "sale
d. "to sale,"

12. The class just finished reading _____________________ a short story by Carl Stephenson about a plantation owner's battle with army ants.

a. -"Leinengen versus the Ants,"
b. Leinengen versus the Ants,
c. "Leinengen versus the Ants,"
d. Leinengen versus the Ants

13. After the car was fixed, it ____________ again.

a. ran good
b. ran well
c. would have run well
d. ran more well

14. "Where does the sun go during the ____________ asked little Kathy.

a. night,"
b. night?",
c. night,?"
d. night?"

15. When I was a child, my mother taught me to say thank you, holding the door open for other, and cover my mouth when yawning or coughing.

a. When I was a child, my mother teaching me to say thank you, to hold the door open for others, and cover my mouth when yawning or coughing.
b. When I was a child, my mother taught me say thank you, to hold the door open for others, and to covering my mouth when yawning or coughing.
c. When I was a child, my mother taught me saying thank you, holding the door open for others, and to cover my mouth when yawning or coughing.
d. When I was a child, my mother taught me to say thank you, hold the door open for others, and cover my mouth when yawning or coughing.

16. Mother is talking to a man that wants to hire her to be a receptionist.

a. Mother is talking to a man who wants to hire her to be a receptionist.

b. Mother is talked to a man who wants to hire her to be a receptionist.

c. Mother is talking to a man who wants to her. To be a receptionist.

d. Mother is talking to a man hiring her who to be a receptionist.

17. Those comic books, which was for sale at the magazine shop, are now quite valuable.

a. Those comics books which were for sale, at the magazine shop are now quite valuable.

b. Those comic books, which were for sale at the magazine, shop, are now quite valuable.

c. Those comic books, which were for sale at the magazine shop, are now, quite valuable

d. Those comic books, which were for sale at the magazine shop, are now quite valuable.

18. If you want to sell your car, it's important being honest with the buyer.

a. If you want to sell your car, being honest with the buyer is important.

b. If you want to sell your car, to be honest with the buyer is important.

c. If you wanting to sell your car, being honest with the buyer are important.

d. If you want to selling your car, to be honest with the buyer is important.

19. Although today the boy was nice to my brother, they usually was quite mean to him.

a. Although today the boy was nice to my brother, they were usually quite mean to him.

b. Although today the boy was nice to my brother, he was usually quite mean to him.

c. Although today the boy were nice to my brother, he is usually quite mean to him.

d. Although today the boy was nice to my brother, he were usually quite mean to him.

Combine the Separate Sentences into one Simpler Sentence with the Same Meaning.

20. The customers were impatient for the store to open. The customers rushed inside as soon as the doors were open.

a. Although the customers were impatient for the store to open, the doors were opened as soon as the customers rushed inside.

b. Although the doors were opened before customers rushed inside, the customers were impatient for the store to open.

c. The customers, who were impatient for the store to open, rushed inside as soon as the doors were open.

d. Although the doors were opened by impatient customers, they rushed inside before the store was open.

21. I should enter my dog in a dog pageant. Everyone says that my dog, whose name is Skipper, is the most beautiful one they've ever seen."

a. Because my dog's name is Skipper, my dog was entered in the pageant and everyone said he was the mot beautiful dog that they've ever seen.

b. I should enter my dog in a dog pageant, since everyone says that Skipper is the most beautiful dog they've ever seen.

c. Before I entered my dog in the dog pageant, Skipper said that he was the most beautiful dog that he'd ever seen.

d. Skipper entered my dog in the dog pageant because he was the most beautiful one that anyone had ever seen.

22. The doctor was not looking forward to meeting Mrs. Lucas. The doctor would have to tell Mrs. Lucas that she has cancer. The doctor hated giving bad news to patients.

a. The doctor hated giving bad news, and so he was not looking forward to meeting Mrs. Lucas because he would have to tell her that she has cancer.

b. The doctor has cancer and was not looking forward to meeting Mrs. Lucas and telling her this bad news.

c. Before the doctor met Mrs. Lucas, he had to give his the patients the bad news that Mrs. Lucas has cancer.

d. The doctor was not looking forward to giving the bad news to his patients that he had to tell Mrs. Lucas that his patients have cancer.

23. Mom hates shopping. We were out of bread, milk and eggs. Mom went to the supermarket.

a. Because we were out of bread, milk and eggs, Mom hated shopping at the supermarket.

b. Although she hates shopping, Mom went to the supermarket since we were out of bread, milk and eggs.

c. Although we were out of bread, milk and eggs, Mom still hated shopping at the supermarket and went there anyway.

d. Because Mom hated shopping at the supermarket, she went to there to buy her bread, milk and eggs.

24. I hate needles. I want to give blood. I can't give blood.

a. Although I hate needles, I can't give blood even if I wanted to.

b. Because I hate needles, I can't give blood, although I want to.

c. Whenever I hate needles, I give blood although I can't give blood.

d. Whenever I can't give blood, I give blood anyway, although I hate needles.

Section IV - Critical Thinking

1. Which word does not belong with the others?

a. Kite

b. Jet

c. Float plane

d. Biplane

2. Which of the following does not belong?

a. Denominate

b. Number

c. Figure

d. Numerate

3. Which of the following does not belong?

a. Abc
b. Nmo
c. Pqr
d. bCD

4. Select the option with the same relationship as Nest : Bird

a. Cave : bear
b. Flower : Petal
c. Window : House
d. Dog : Basket

5. Select the option with the same relationship as Teacher : School

a. Fish : Water
b. Waitress : Coffee shop
c. Dentist : Tooth
d. Businessman : Money

6. Select the option with the same relationship as Pebble : Boulder

a. Fish : Elephant
b. River: Rapids
c. Pond : Ocean
d. Feather : Bird

7. Select the option with the same relationship as Poodle : Dog

a. Shark : Great White
b. Dalmatian : Great Dane
c. Money : Stock Market
d. Horse : Pony

8. Consider the following series: 6, 12, 24, 48, ... What number should come next?

a. 60
b. 64
c. 48
d. 96

9. Consider the following series: 5, 6, 11, 17, ... What number should come next?

a. 34
b. 36
c. 28
d. 27

10. Consider the following series: 26, 21, __ , 11, 6. What is the missing number?

a. 16
b. 29
c. 23
d. 27

11. Which of the following does not belong?

a. CD
b. OP
c. LM
d. BD

12. Which of the following does not belong?

a. 151415
b. 121212
c. 141414
d. 292929

13. Which of the following does not belong?

a. 246
b. 468
c. 123
d. 024

14. Select the option with the same relationship as fox : chicken

a. cat : mouse
b. rat : mouse
c. dog : cat
d. rabbit : hen

15. Select the option with the same relationship as lawyer : trial

a. plumber : pipe
b. businessman : secretary
c. doctor : operation
d. hairdresser : blow dryer

16. Select the option with the same relationship as Wax : Candle

a. Clay : bowl
b. Ink : pen
c. String : Kite
d. Liquid : Cup

17. Consider the following series: 25, 33, 41, 49, ... What number should come next?

a. 59
b. 55
c. 51
d. 57

18. Consider the following series: 6, 11, 18, 27, ... What number should come next?

a. 35
b. 38
c. 29
d. 30

19. Consider the following series: 13, 26, 52, 104, ... What number should come next?

a. 106
b. 200
c. 400
d. 208

20. Consider the following series: 32, 26, 20, 14, ... What number should come next?

a. 8
b. 10
c. 19
d. 12

Section IV – Basic Science

1. Which, if any, of the following statements about the respiratory system are true?

a. The respiratory system consists of all the organs involved in breathing.
b. Organs included in the respiratory system are the nose, pharynx, larynx, trachea, bronchi and lungs.
c. The respiratory system conveys oxygen into our bodies and removes carbon dioxide from our bodies.
d. All of the Above.

2. The ________ system maintains the body's balance through the release of ________ directly into the bloodstream.

a. The gastrointestinal system maintains the body's balance through the release of hormones directly into the bloodstream.
b. The endocrine system maintains the body's balance through the release of oxygen directly into the bloodstream.
c. The digestive system maintains the body's balance through the release of hormones directly into the bloodstream.
d. The endocrine system maintains the body's balance through the release of hormones directly into the bloodstream.

3. Among others, the endocrine system includes:

a. The pituitary gland
b. The thyroid gland
c. The adrenal glands
d. All of the Above.

4. _______ are contractile organs that cause movement when stimulated; the three types are _____, _____, and ______.

a. Muscles are expansion organs that cause movement when stimulated; the three types are smooth, cardiac, and skeletal.

b. Muscles are contractile organs that cause movement when stimulated; the three types are smooth, cardiac, and skeletal.

c. Muscles are contractile organs that cause movement when stimulated; the three types are semipermeable, cardiac, and skeletal.

d. Muscles are contractile organs that cause movement when stimulated; the three types are respiratory, cardiac, and skeletal.

5. Which of the following is not a function of the skeletal system?

a. Providing the shape and form of our bodies

b. Supporting and protecting the body

c. Producing Blood

d. Storing vitamins

6. What is the number of bones included in the human skeletal system?

a. 412

b. 103

c. Over 300

d. 206

7. ______ are connected to ___ by _____, and _____ are connected to each other by _____.

a. Muscles are connected to bones by tendons, and bones are connected to each other by ligaments.

b. Tendons are connected to bones by ligaments, and bones are connected to each other by tendons.

c. Muscles are connected to bones by ligaments, and bones are connected to each other by tendons.

d. Ligaments are connected to bones by tendons, and bones are connected to each other by bands.

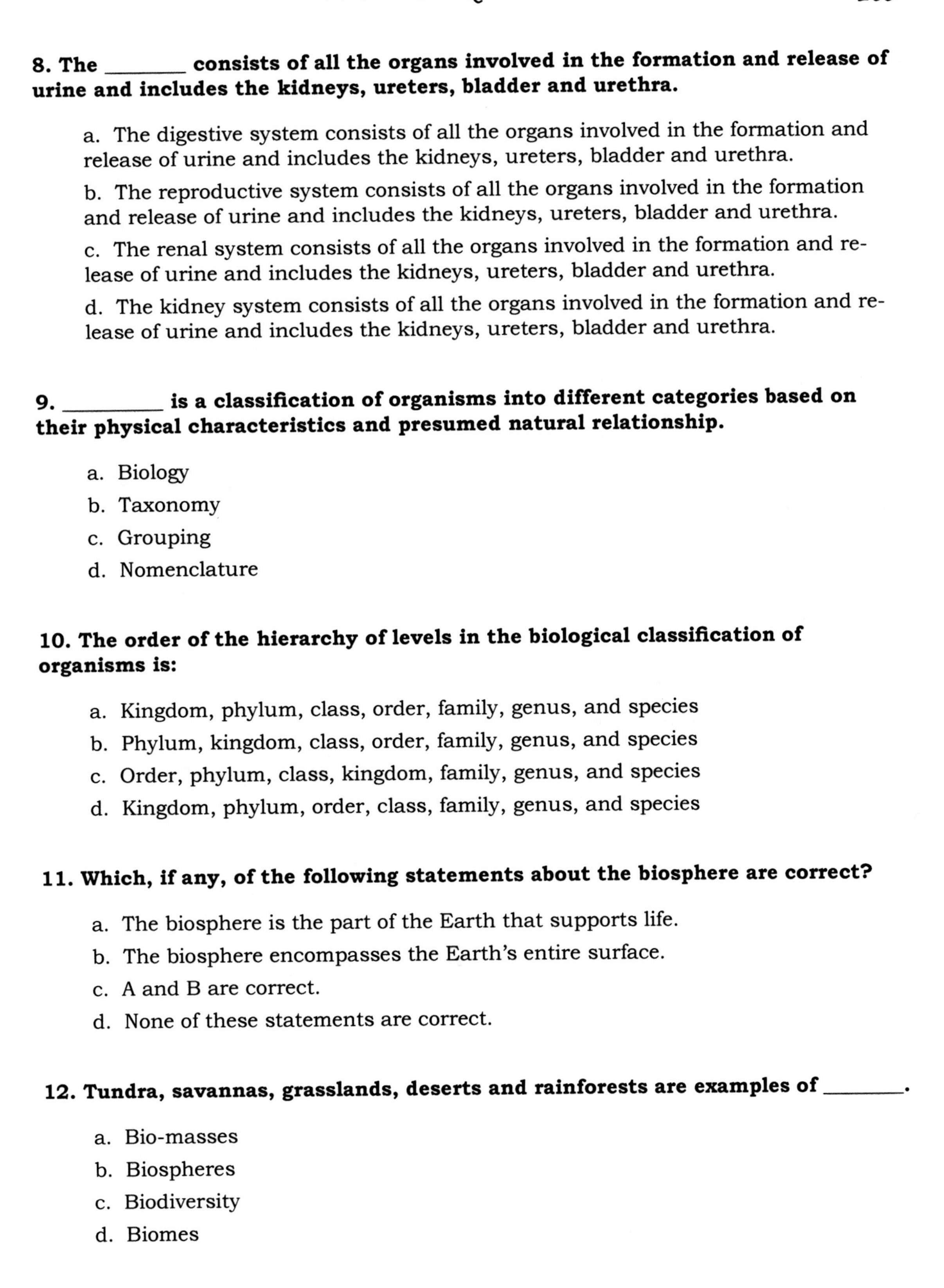

8. The _______ consists of all the organs involved in the formation and release of urine and includes the kidneys, ureters, bladder and urethra.

a. The digestive system consists of all the organs involved in the formation and release of urine and includes the kidneys, ureters, bladder and urethra.

b. The reproductive system consists of all the organs involved in the formation and release of urine and includes the kidneys, ureters, bladder and urethra.

c. The renal system consists of all the organs involved in the formation and release of urine and includes the kidneys, ureters, bladder and urethra.

d. The kidney system consists of all the organs involved in the formation and release of urine and includes the kidneys, ureters, bladder and urethra.

9. _________ is a classification of organisms into different categories based on their physical characteristics and presumed natural relationship.

a. Biology

b. Taxonomy

c. Grouping

d. Nomenclature

10. The order of the hierarchy of levels in the biological classification of organisms is:

a. Kingdom, phylum, class, order, family, genus, and species

b. Phylum, kingdom, class, order, family, genus, and species

c. Order, phylum, class, kingdom, family, genus, and species

d. Kingdom, phylum, order, class, family, genus, and species

11. Which, if any, of the following statements about the biosphere are correct?

a. The biosphere is the part of the Earth that supports life.

b. The biosphere encompasses the Earth's entire surface.

c. A and B are correct.

d. None of these statements are correct.

12. Tundra, savannas, grasslands, deserts and rainforests are examples of _______.

a. Bio-masses

b. Biospheres

c. Biodiversity

d. Biomes

13. The mixture of gases surrounding a planet is its ______________.

a. Atmosphere
b. Stratosphere
c. Biosphere
d. Troposphere

14. In order, from lower to upper, the layers of the atmosphere are:

a. Exosphere, thermosphere, mesosphere, stratosphere, troposphere
b. Troposphere, stratosphere, mesosphere, thermosphere, exosphere
c. Mesosphere, troposphere, stratosphere, , thermosphere, exosphere
d. Thermosphere, troposphere, stratosphere, mesosphere, , exosphere

15. The force per unit area exerted against a surface by the weight of air above that surface in the Earth's atmosphere is the _________ _________.

a. Gravitational force
b. Atmospheric pressure
c. Barometric density
d. Aneroid pressure

16. Which, if any, of the following statements are true?

a. Water boils at approximately 100 °C (212 °F) at standard atmospheric pressure.
b. The boiling point is the temperature at which the vapor pressure is higher than the atmospheric pressure around the water.
c. Water boils at a lower temperature in areas of lower pressure.
d. A and C are true.

17. ___ _________ ______ is the effect of the Earth's rotation on the atmosphere and on all objects on the Earth's surface.

a. The Coriolis effect
b. The Corona effect
c. The Archimedes effect
d. The tidal effect

18. Binding membrane of an animal cell is called,

a. Biological membrane
b. Cell coat
c. Unit membrane
d. Plasma membrane

19. The segment of a DNA molecule that determines the amino acid sequence of protein is known as ____?

a. Operator gene
b. Structural gene
c. Regulator gene
d. Modifier gene

20. Cells that line the inner or outer surfaces of organs or body cavities are often linked together by intimate physical connections. These connections are referred to as____

a. Separate desmosomes
b. Ronofilaments
c. Tight junctions
d. Fascia adherenes

21. Which one of the following best describes the function of a cell membrane?

a. It controls the substances entering and leaving the cell.
b. It keeps the cell in shape.
c. It controls the substances entering the cell.
d. It supports the cell structures

22. Which of the following arrangement is seen in the plasma membrane?

a. Lipids with embedded proteins
b. An outer lipid layer and an inner lipid layer
c. Proteins embedded in lipid bilayer
d. Altering protein and lipid layers

23. Genes control heredity in man and other organisms. This gene is ____

a. A segment of DNA

b. A bead like structure on the chromosomes

c. A protein molecule

d. A segment of RNA

24. A(an) _______ _______ is a description of a _______ _______ that gives the chemical formulas of the reactants and the_______ of the reaction, with coefficients introduced so that the number of each type of atom and the total charge is _______ by the reaction.

a. A balanced comparison is a description of a biological reaction that gives the chemical formulas of the reactants and the consequences of the reaction, with coefficients introduced so that the number of each type of atom and the total charge is unchanged by the reaction.

b. A reactant chemical equation is a description of a chemical reaction that gives the chemical formulas of the reactants and the products of the reaction, with coefficients introduced so that the number of each type of atom and the total charge is unchanged by the reaction.

c. A balanced equation is a description of a chemical reaction that gives the chemical formulas of the reactants and the products of the reaction, with coefficients introduced so that the number of each type of atom and the total charge is changed by the reaction.

d. A balanced equation is a description of a chemical reaction that gives the chemical formulas of the reactants and the products of the reaction, with coefficients introduced so that the number of each type of atom and the total charge is unchanged by the reaction.

25. _______ bonds involve a complete sharing of electrons and occurs most commonly between atoms that have partially filled outer shells or energy levels.

a. Covalent

b. Ionic

c. Hydrogen

d. Proportional

26. The reaction of elements with low electronegativity(almost empty outer shells) with elements with high electronegativity (mostly full outer shells) gives rise to _______ bonds.

a. Hydrogen

b. Covalent

c. Ionic

d. Nuclear

27. _________ bonds involve electrons that are not equally shared, and may be deemed as an intermediate between the extremes represented by _______ and ________ bonds.

a. Ionic bonds involve electrons that are not equally shared, and may be deemed as an intermediate between the extremes represented by covalent and polar bonds.

b. Covalent bonds involve electrons that are not equally shared, and may be deemed as an intermediate between the extremes represented by polar and ionic bonds.

c. Chemical bonds involve electrons that are not equally shared, and may be deemed as an intermediate between the extremes represented by covalent and ionic bonds.

d. Polar bonds involve electrons that are not equally shared, and may be deemed as an intermediate between the extremes represented by covalent and ionic bonds.

28. __________ _______ involve an especially strong dipole-dipole force between molecules, and are responsible for the unique properties of water and pin DNA into its characteristic shape.

a. Oxygen links
b. Hydrogen bonds
c. Nitrogen bonds
d. Dipolar bonds

29. _______________ predicts that the solubility (C) of a gas or volatile substance in a liquid is proportional to the partial pressure (P) of the substance over the liquid (P = k C).

a. Boyle's law
b. Gay-Lussac's Law
c. Henry's law
d. Charles' law

30. ___________ states that the pressure of an ideal gas is inversely proportional to its volume, if the temperature and amount of gas are held constant.

a. Henry's law
b. Dalton's law
c. Brown's law
d. Boyle's law

31. Which of the following statements, if any, are correct?

a. pH is a measure of effective concentration of hydrogen ions in a solution, and is approximately related to the molarity of H+ by pH = - log [H+]

b. pH is a measure of effective concentration of oxygen ions in a solution, and is approximately related to the molarity of O+ by pH = - log [O+]

c. pH is a measure of effective concentration of hydrogen atoms in a solution, and is approximately related to the polarity of H+ by pH = - log [H+]

d. Acidity is a measure of effective concentration of hydrogen ions in a solution, and is approximately related to the molarity of H+ by pH = - log [H+]

32. Four factors that affect rates of reaction are:

a. Barometric pressure, particle size, concentration, and the presence of a facilitator

b. Temperature, particle size, concentration, and the presence of a catalyst

c. Temperature, container material, elevation, and the presence of instability

d. Volatility, particle size, concentration, and the presence of a catalyst

33. One factor that affects rates of reaction is concentration. Which of these statements about concentration is/are correct?

a. A higher concentration of reactants causes more effective collisions per unit time, leading to an increased reaction rate.

b. A lower concentration of reactants causes more effective collisions per unit time, leading to an increased reaction rate.

c. A higher concentration of reactants causes more effective collisions per unit time, leading to a decreased reaction rate.

d. A higher concentration of reactants causes less effective collisions per unit time, leading to an increased reaction rate.

34. ____________ is expressed by the equation: $P_{tot} = P_a + P_b$, whereby P is pressure, P_{tot} is total pressure, P_a and P_b are component pressures.

a. Henry's law

b. Dalton's law

c. Boyle's law

d. Gay-Lussac's law

35. A/an _________ is an element with both metallic and non-metallic properties. Examples are silicon, arsenic, and germanium.

a. Metalloid
b. Conglomerate
c. Semi-metal
d. Amalgamate

36. Which, if any, of these statements about solubility are correct?

a. The solubility of a substance is its concentration in a saturated solution.
b. Substances with solubilities much less than 1 g/ 100 mL of solvent are usually considered insoluble.
c. A saturated solution is one which does not dissolve any more solute.
d. All of these statements are correct.

37. Which, if any, of the following statements are false?

a. In an endothermic process, solubility increases with the increase in temperature and decreases if the temperature decreases.
b. In an exothermic process, solubility decreases with an increase in temperature.
c. All of the Above.
d. None of the Above.

38. ____________ is the spontaneous, random movement of small particles suspended in liquid, caused by the unbalanced impacts of molecules on the particle.

a. Brownian motion
b. Grey's kinesis
c. Boyle's wave
d. None of the above

39. _________ is defined as the number of cycles of a wave that move past a fixed observation point per second.

a. Wave
b. Wavelength
c. Frequency
d. Wave function

40. __________ is defined as the distance between adjacent peaks (or adjacent troughs) on a wave.

a. Frequency
b. Wavenumber
c. Wave oscillation
d. Wavelength

41. ______________ is a mathematical function that gives the amplitude of a wave as a function of position (and sometimes, as a function of time and/or electron spin).

a. Wavelength
b. Frequency
c. Wavenumber
d. Wavefunction

42. In the periodic table the elements are arranged in

a. Order of increasing atomic number
b. Alphabetical order
c. Order of increasing metallic properties
d. Order of increasing neutron content

43. A molecule of water contains hydrogen and oxygen in a 1:8 ratio by mass. This is a statement of ________.

a. The law of multiple proportions
b. The law of conservation of mass
c. The law of conservation of energy
d. The law of constant composition

44. Different isotopes of a particular element contain the same number of _________.

a. Protons
b. Neutrons
c. Protons and neutrons
d. Protons, neutrons and electrons

45. The s block and p block elements are collectively known as _____?

a. Transition elements
b. Active elements
c. Representative elements
d. Inactive elements

46. Who was the English scientist who made accurate observations on how pressure and volume are related?

a. Charles
b. Combine
c. Boyle
d. Gay-Lussac

47. When pressure on a gas is reduced to half what happens to its volume?

a. The volume stays the same
b. The volume decreases
c. The volume rises then falls
d. The volume increases

48. What is the standard temperature in Kelvin?

a. 25 Kelvin
b. 273 Kelvin
c. 0 kelvin
d. 373 Kelvin

49. Real gases approach ideal behavior under which of the following conditions?

a. At high pressure and high temperature
b. At low pressure and high temperature
c. Near the boiling point of water
d. Real gases can never exhibit ideal behavior

50. The temperature and volume of a gas are directly related. This is a statement of:

a. Combined Gas Law

b. Boyle's Law

c. Charles' Law

d. The Ideal Gas Law

Answer Key

1. B
We can infer an important part of the respiratory system are the lungs. From the passage, "Molecules of oxygen and carbon dioxide are passively exchanged, by diffusion, between the gaseous external environment and the blood. This exchange process occurs in the alveolar region of the lungs."

Therefore, one primary function for the respiratory system is the exchange of oxygen and carbon dioxide, and this process occurs in the lungs. We can therefore infer that the lungs are an important part of the respiratory system.

2. C
The process by which molecules of oxygen and carbon dioxide are passively exchanged is diffusion.

This is a definition type question. Scan the passage for references to "oxygen," "carbon dioxide," or "exchanged."

3. A
The organ that plays an important role in gas exchange in amphibians is the skin.

Scan the passage for references to "amphibians," and find the answer.

4. A
The three physiological zones of the respiratory system are Conducting, transitional, respiratory zones.

5. A
Secede most nearly means to break away from because the 11 states wanted to leave the United States and form their own country.

Option B is incorrect because the states were not accomplishing anything
Option C is incorrect because the states were trying to leave the USA not join it. Option D is incorrect because the states seceded before they lost the war.

6. B
Look at the dates in the passage. The shots were fired on April 12 and Congress declared war on April 14.

Option A is incorrect because the dates show clearly which happened first. Option C is incorrect because the passage states that Lincoln was against slavery. Option D is incorrect because it never mentions who was or was not at Fort Sumter.

7. C
The passage clearly states that Lee surrendered to Grant after the capture of the capital of the Confederacy, which is Richmond. A is incorrect because the war continued for 2 years after Gettysburg.

Option B is incorrect because that battle is never mentioned in the passage. Option D is incorrect because the capture of the capital occurred after the march to the sea.

8. A
When the passage said that the North had abolished slavery, it implies that slaves were no longer allowed to be had in the North. In essence slavery was banned.

Option B is incorrect because it makes no sense relative to the context of the passage. Option C is incorrect because we know the North was fighting slavery, not for it. Option D is incorrect because slavery is not a tangible thing that can be destroyed. It is a practice that had to be outlawed or banned.

9. B
The first paragraph tells us that myths are a true account of the remote past.

The second paragraph tells us that, "myths generally take place during a primordial age, when the world was still young, before achieving its current form."

Putting these two together, we can infer that humankind used myth to explain how the world was created.

10. A
This passage is about different types of stories. First, the passage explains myths, and then compares other types of stories to myths.

11. B
From the passage, "Unlike myths, folktales can take place at any time and any place, and the natives do not usually consider them true or sacred."

12. A
Based on the partial table of contents, this book is most likely about how to answer multiple choice.

13. B
This passage describes the different categories for traditional stories. The other options are facts from the passage, not the main idea of the passage. The main idea of a passage will always be the most general statement. For example, Option A, Myths, fables, and folktales are not the same thing, and each describes a specific type of story. This is a true statement from the passage, but not the main idea of the passage, since the passage also talks about how some cultures may classify a story as a myth and others as a folktale.

The statement, from Option B, Traditional stories can be categorized in different ways by different people, is a more general statement that describes the passage.

14. B
Option B is the best choice, categories that group traditional stories according to certain characteristics.

Options A and C are false and can be eliminated right away. Option D is designed to confuse. Option D may be true, but it is not mentioned in the passage.

15. D
The best answer is D, traditional stories themselves are a part of the larger category of folklore, which may also include costumes, gestures, and music.

All the other options are false. Traditional stories are part of the larger category of Folklore, which includes other things, not the other way around.

16. A
There is a distinct difference between a myth and a legend, although, both are folktales.

17. C
To be infamous means to be remembered for an evil or terrible action. Therefore, the word infamy means to remember a bad or terrible thing.

Option A is incorrect because being famous is not the same as being infamous. Option D is incorrect because Pearl Harbor was not forgotten.

18. C
Each other answer set contains the name of at least one country who was not part of the AXIS powers.

19. D
The answer is stated directly in the passage.

Option A is in correct because there was no indication that Japan would attack San Diego. Option B is incorrect because the attack on Pearl Harbor was a surprise. Option C is incorrect because Roosevelt was not planning to attack Japan.

20. C
The passage clearly states that Japan planned a surprise attack. They chose that early time in order to catch the U.S. military off guard. Option A is incorrect because the military does not sleep late. Option B is incorrect because there is no law against bombing countries. Option D is incorrect because it makes no sense.

21. B

This question tests the reader's summarization skills. A is a very broad statement that may or may not be true, and seems to be in context, but has nothing to do with the passage. The author does mention that the statue was probably used on a temple dedicated to the Greek gods (D), but in no way discusses or argues for the gods' attitude toward, or claim on these temples or its faucets. Nike does indeed lead the gods into a war (the Titan war), as option C suggests, but this is not mentioned by the passage and students who know this may be drawn to this answer but have not done a close enough analysis of the text that is actually in the passage. Option B is appropriately expository, and connects the titular emphasis to the idea that the Greek gods are very important to Greek culture.

22. C

This question tests the reader's summarization skills. The test for question option C is pulled straight from the paragraph, but is not word-for-word, so it may seem too obvious to be the right answer. The passage does talk about Nike being the goddess of war, as A states, but the third paragraph only touches on it and it is an inference that soldiers destroyed the statue, when this question is asking specifically for what the third paragraph actually stated. Option B is also straight from the text, with a minor but key change: the inclusion of the words "all" and "never" are too limiting and the passage does not suggest that these limits exist. If a reader selects option D, they are also making an inference that is misguided for this type of question. The paragraph does state that the arms and head are "lost" but does not suggest who lost them.

23. A

This question tests the reader's ability to recognize function in writing. Option B can be eliminated based on the purpose of the passage, which is expository and not persuasive. The author may or may not feel this way, but the passage does not show evidence of being argumentative for that purpose. Options C and D are both details found in the text, but, neither of them encompasses the entire message of the passage, which has an overall message of learning about culture from art and making guesses about how the two are related, as suggested by option A.

24. D

This question tests the reader's ability to understand function within writing. Most of the possible selections are very general statements which may or may not be true. It probably is a student who is taking the test on which this question is featured (A), but the author makes no address to the test taker and is not talking to the audience in terms of the test. Likewise, it may also be true that students read more than adults (C), mandated by schools and grades, but the focus on the verb "read" in the first sentence is too narrow and misses the larger purpose of the passage; the same could be said for option B. While all the statements could be true, option D is the most germane, and infers the purpose of the passage without making assumptions that could be incorrect.

25. B

The time limit for radar detectors is 14 days. Since you made the purchase 15 days ago, you do not qualify for the guarantee.

26. B

Since you made the purchase 10 days ago, the guarantee covers you. Since it is an advertised price at a different store, ABC Electric will "beat" the price by 10% of the difference, which is,

500 – 400 = 100 – difference in price

100 X 10% = $10 – 10% of the difference

The advertised lower price is $400. ABC will beat this price by 10% so they will refund $100 + 10 = $110.

27. C
The purpose of this passage is to persuade.

28. D
This question tests the reader's summarization skills. The question is asking very generally about the message of the passage, and the title, "Ways Characters Communicate in Theater," is one indication of that. The other options A, B, and C are all directly from the text, and therefore readers may be inclined to select one of them, but are too specific to encapsulate the entirety of the passage and its message.

29. B
The paragraph on soliloquies mentions "To be or not to be," and it is from the context of that paragraph that readers may understand that because "To be or not to be" is a soliloquy, Hamlet will be introspective, or thoughtful, while delivering it. It is true that actors deliver soliloquies alone, and may be "solitary" (A), but "thoughtful" (B) is more true to the overall idea of the paragraph. Readers may choose option C because drama and theater can be used interchangeably and the passage mentions that soliloquies are unique to theater (and therefore drama), but this answer is not specific enough to the paragraph in question. Readers may pick up on the theme of life and death and Hamlet's true intentions and select that he is "hopeless" (D), but those themes are not discussed either by this paragraph or passage, as a close textual reading and analysis confirms.

30. C
This question tests the reader's grammatical skills. Option B seems logical, but parenthesis are actually considered to be a stronger break in a sentence than commas are, and along this line of thinking, actually disrupt the sentence more. Options A and D make comparisons between theater and film that are simply not made in the passage, and may or may not be true. This detail does clarify the statement that asides are most unique to theater by adding that it is not completely unique to theater, which may have been why the author didn't chose not to delete it and instead used parentheses to designate the detail's importance (C).

31. C
This question tests the reader's vocabulary and contextualization skills. A may or may not be true, but focuses on the wrong function of the word "give" and ignores the rest of the sentence, which is more relevant to what the passage is discussing. Options B and D may also be selected if the reader depends too literally on the word "give," failing to grasp the more abstract function of the word that is the focus of option C, which also properly acknowledges the entirety of the passage and its meaning.

32. A
We can infer that an important purpose of the circulatory system is that of fighting diseases.

33. B
Humans have a closed circulatory system.

34. C
In addition to blood, the heart and the blood vessels form the cardiovascular system.

35. B
The digestive system, along with the circulatory system, helps provide nutrients to keep the human heart pumping.

36. A
We can infer that blood is responsible for transporting oxygen to the cells.

37. A
Human blood cells suspended in plasma.

38. C
Calcium is not contained in blood plasma.

From the passage, "[Blood Plasma] contains dissolved proteins, glucose, mineral ions, hormones, carbon dioxide, platelets and the blood cells themselves."

39. A
The lungs exhale the carbon dioxide after venous blood has been carried from body tissues.

40. A
The main idea of this passage is that the human skeleton is an important and complicated system of the body.

We can infer the skeleton is important because it protects important organs like brain, lungs and heart. We know the skeleton is complicated because it consists of a number of parts, (ligaments, tendons, muscles and cartilage) and 206 bones.

This general statement best describes the passage. The other choices are details mentioned in the passage.

Section II - Math

1. D
8327 – 1278 = 7049

2. B
294 X 21 = 6174

3. C
1278 + 4920 = 6198

4. A
285 * 12 = 3420

5. C
4120 – 3216 = 904

6. D
2417 + 1004 = 3421

7. B
1440 ÷ 12 = 120

8. C
2713 – 1308 = 1405

9. D
$x^2 + 4x = 5$, $x^2 + 4x - 5 = 0$, $x^2 + 5x - x - 5 = 0$, factorize $x(x+5) - 1(x+5) = o$, $(x+5)(x-1)=0$. $x + 5 = 0$ or $x - 1 = 0$, $x = 0 - 5$ or $x = 0 + 1$, $x = -5$ or $x = 1$, either b or c.

10. C
Open parenthesis: $2a + 2b = 4ab$, divide both sides by $2 = a+b=2ab$ or $a+b=ab + ab$, therefore $a=ab$ and $b=ab$, therefore $a=b$.

11. B
Let the XY represent the initial number, X + Y = 12, YX=XY+ 36, Only b = 48 satisfies both equations above from the given options.

12. A

13. B
Let the father's age=Y, and Kate's age=X, therefore Y=32+X, in 5yrs y=5x,substituting for Y will be 5x = 32+X, 5x – x = 32, 4X=32,X= 32/8, x = 8, Kate will be 8 in 5 years time, so Kate's present age = 8 - 5 = 3.

14. A
This is a simple direct proportion problem: If Lynn can type 1 page in p minutes,

She can type x pages in 5 minutes

We do cross multiplication: $x \cdot p = 5 \cdot 1$

Then,

$x = 5/p$

15. A
This is an inverse ration problem.

$1/x = 1/a + 1/b$ where a is the time Sally can paint a house, b is the time John can paint a house, x is the time Sally and John can together paint a house.

So,

1/x = 1/4 + 1/6 ... We use the least common multiple in the denominator that is 24:

1/x = 6/24 + 4/24

1/x = 10/24

x = 24/10

x = 2.4 hours.

In other words; 2 hours + 0.4 hours = 2 hours + 0.4•60 minutes

= 2 hours 24 minutes

16. D
The cost of the dishwasher = $450

15% discount amount = 450•15/100 = $67.5

The discounted price = 450 – 67.5 = $382.5

20% additional discount amount on lowest price = 382.5•20/100 = $76.5

So, the final discounted price = 382.5 - 76.5 = $306.00

17. D
Original price = x,
80/100 = 12590/X,
80X = 1259000,
X = 15737.50.

18. C
Total hay = 214 kg,
The goat eats at a rate of 214/60days = 3.6kg per day.
The Cow eats at a rate of 214/15 = 14.3kg per day,
Together they eat 3.6 + 14.3 = 17.9 per day.
At a rate of 17.9kg per day, they will consume 214kg in 214/17.9 = 11.96 or 12 days approx.

19. A
25% = 25/100 = 1/4

20. C
125/100 = 1.25

21. D
40/100 = 30/X = 40X = 30*100 = 3000/40 = 75

22. B
12.5/100 = 50/X = 12.5X = 50 * 100 = 5000/12.5 = 400

23. C
24/56 = 3/7 (divide numerator and denominator by 8)

24. C
Converting percent to decimal – divide percent by 100 and remove the % sign. 87% = 87/100 = .87

25. A
60 has the same relation to X as 75 to 100 – so
60/X = 75/100
6000 = 75X
X = 80

26. D
60 has the same relationship to 100 as 12 does to X – so
60/100 = 12/X
1200 = 60X
X = 20

27. C
Converting a fraction into a decimal – divide the numerator by the denominator – so 71/1000 = .071. Dividing by 1000 moves the decimal point 3 places.

28. C
4.7 + .9 + .01 = 5.61

29. A
.33 × .59 = .1947

30. D
.84 ÷ .7 = 1.2

31. C
9 is in the ten thousandths place in 1.7389.

32. A
.87 - .48 = .39

33. A
Step 1: Set up the formula to calculate the dose to be given in mg as per weight of the child:-
Dose ordered X Weight in Kg = Dose to be given
Step 2: 100 mg X 23 kg = 2300 mg
(Convert 50 lb to Kg, 1 lb = 0.4536 kg, hence 50 lb = 50 X 0.4536 = 22.68 kg approx. 23 kg)
2300 mg/230 mg X 1 tablet/1 = 2300/230 = 10 tablets

34. B
1000 units/5000 units X 1 ml/1 = 1000/5000 = 0.2 ml

35. C
4 x 4 x 4 = 64

36. D
5 ml/15 ml kX 1 tsp/1 = 5/15 = 0.3 tsp

37. B
70 mg/1000 mg X 1 ml/1 = 70/1000 – 0.07 ml
(Convert 1 g = 1000 mg)

38. C
200 mg/400 mg X 1 tsp/1 = 200/400 = 0.5 tsp

39. D
600 mg/ 200 mg X 1 tablet/1 = 600/200 = 3 tablets

40. A
At 100% efficiency 1 machine produces 1450/10 = 145 m of cloth.

At 95% efficiency, 4 machines produce 4•145•95/100 = 551 m of cloth.

At 90% efficiency, 6 machines produce 6•145•90/100 = 783 m of cloth.

Total cloth produced by all 10 machines = 551 + 783 = 1334 m

Since the information provided and the question are based on 8 hours, we did not need to use time to reach the answer.

41. C
1 foot = 12 inches, 60 feet = 60 x 12 = 720 inches.

42. A
1 centimeter = 10 millimeter, 25 centimeter = 25 X 10 = 250.

43. A
1 millimeter = 10 centimeters, 100 millimeter = 100/10 = 10 centimeters.

44. C
1 gallon = 4 quarts, 3 gallons = 3 x 4 = 12 quarts.

45. A
There are 1000 mm in a meter.

46. B
There are 1000 ml in a liter. 0.05/1000 = 0.00005 liters.

47. D
There are 1000 mg in a gram. 30/1000 = 0.03 grams.

48. A
There are 10 mm in a cm. 0.101/10 = .0101

49. B
The formula of the volume of cylinder is the base area multiplied by the height. As the formula:

Volume of a cylinder = $\pi r^2 h$. Where π is 3.142, r is radius of the cross sectional area, and h is the height.

We know that the diameter is 5 meters, so

the radius is 5/2 = 2.5 meters.

The volume is: $V = 3.142 \cdot 2.5^2 \cdot 12 = 235.65$ m^3.

50. B
There are 52 cards in total. Smith has 16 cards in which he can win. Therefore, his probability of winning in a single game will be 16/52. Simon has 20 winning cards so his probability of winning in single draw is 20/52.

Section IV – English Grammar

1. D
The preposition "to" is correct. "To" here means give.

2. A
"Lie" means to recline, and does not take an object. "lay" means to place and does take an object.

3. A
Past unreal conditional. Takes the form, [If ... Past Perfect ..., ... would have + past participle ...]

4. B
This sentence is in the present tense, so "to find" is correct.

5. B
The comma separates a phrase.

6. A
Possessive pronouns ending in s take an apostrophe before the 's': one's; everyone's; somebody's, nobody else's, etc.

7. D
When talking about something that didn't happen in the past, use the past perfect (if I had done).

8. C
"Lie" means to recline, and does not take an object. "Lay" means to place and does take an object. Peter lay the books on the table (the books are the direct object), or the telephone poles were lying on the road (no direct object).

9. A
Titles of short stories are enclosed in quotation marks.

10. C
No additional punctuation is required here.

11. B
Here the word "sale" is used as a "word" and not as a word in the sentence, so quotation marks are used.

12. C
Titles of short stories are enclosed in quotation marks, and commas always go inside quotation marks.

13. B
"Ran well" is correct. "Ran good" is never correct.

14. D
Commas and periods always go inside quotation marks. Question marks that are part of a quote also go inside quotation marks; however, if the writer quotes a statement as part of a larger question, the question mark is placed after the quotation mark.

15. D
The sentence starts with a phrase, which is separated by a comma and then lists the things the speaker's mother taught, to say thank you, etc. Each of the items in the list are separated by a comma.

16. A
When referring to a person, use "who" instead of "that."

17. A
The comma separates a phrase starting

with 'which.'

18. A
"Being honest," present tense is the best choice. "The buyer" is singular so use "is."

19. C
The subject in the first phrase, "the boy," has to agree with the subject in the second phrase, "he is."

20. C
These two sentences can be combined into one sentence with 2 clauses separated by a comma.

21. B
These two sentences can be combined and the phrase, 'whose name is Skipper,' deleted.

22. A
These three sentences can be combined using 'although,' and 'even if.'

23. B
These two sentences can be combined into one sentence with two clauses separated by a comma.

24. A
These three sentences can be combined using 'although,' and 'since.'

Section IV - Critical Thinking

1. A
A kite is not a type of plane.

2. C
This is a relationship of words question. All of the choices are synonyms of count, except figure.

3. D
This is a capital small letter relationship. All choices start with a capital letter.

4. A
This is a functional relationship. A Bird lives in a nest, the same way that a bear lives in a cave.

5. B
This is a functional relationship. A teacher works in a school in the same way that a Waitress works in a coffee shop.

6. C
This is a Degree relationship. A boulder is a very large pebble - both are rocks, in the same way an ocean is a very large pond - both are very bodies of water.

7. A
This is a type relationship. A poodle is a type of dog in the same way a great white is a type of shark.

8. D
The numbers doubles each time.

9. C
Each number is the sum of the previous two numbers

10. A
The numbers decrease by 5 each time.

11. D
BD is not a sequence of consecutive letters.

12. A
This is a repetition patter All of the choices repeat a 2-letter sequence.

13. C
123 are consecutive, the others are obtained by adding 2.

14. A
This is a predator/prey relationship. Foxes eat chickens in the same way as cats eat mice.

15. C
This is a functional relationship. A lawyer

defends a client in a trial in the same way that a doctor performs an operation on a patient.

16. A
This is a composition relationship. A candle is made of wax and a bowl is made of clay.

17. D
The numbers increase by 8.

18. B
The interval begins with 5, increases by 2 and is added each time.

19. D
The number doubles each time.

20. A
The numbers decrease by 6 each time.

Section V – Basic Science

1. D
All of the statements are true.

a. The respiratory system consists of all the organs involved in breathing.

b. Organs included in the respiratory system are the nose, pharynx, larynx, trachea, bronchi and lungs.

c. The respiratory system conveys oxygen into our bodies and removes carbon dioxide from our bodies.

2. D
The **endocrine** system maintains the body's balance through the release of **hormones** directly into the bloodstream.

3. D
All of the above. The endocrine system includes:

a. The pituitary gland

b. The thyroid gland

c. The adrenal glands

4. B
Muscles are contractile organs that cause movement when stimulated; the three types are **smooth**, **cardiac**, and **skeletal**.

5. D
Storing vitamins **is not a function of the skeletal system.**

6. D
There are 206 bones in the skeletal system.

7. A
Muscles are connected to **bones** by **tendons**, and **ligaments connect bones to each other**.

8. C
The **renal system** consists of all the organs involved in the formation and release of urine and includes the kidneys, ureters, bladder and urethra.

9. B
Taxonomy is a classification of organisms into different categories based on their physical characteristics and presumed natural relationship.

10. A
The order of the hierarchy of levels in the biological classification of organisms is: **Kingdom, phylum, class, order, family, genus, and species.**

Note: A useful mnemonic device to remember this order is:
"Kids Prefer Cheese Over Fried Green Spinach."

11. A and B are correct.
a. The biosphere is the part of the Earth that supports life.
c. The biosphere is limited to the waters of the Earth, a fraction of its

crust and the lower regions of the atmosphere.

12. D
Tundra, savannas, grasslands, deserts and rainforests are examples of biomes.

13. A
The mixture of gases surrounding a planet is its **atmosphere**.

14. B
In order, from lower to upper, the layers of the atmosphere are:
troposphere, stratosphere, mesosphere, thermosphere, exosphere.

15. B
The force per unit area exerted against a surface by the weight of air above that surface in the Earth's atmosphere is the **atmospheric pressure**.

16. D A and C are correct.
a. Water boils at approximately 100 °C (212 °F) at standard atmospheric pressure.
c. Water boils at a lower temperature in areas of lower pressure.

17. A
The Coriolis effect is the effect of the Earth's rotation on the atmosphere and on all objects on the Earth's surface.

Note: In the northern hemisphere, the Coriolis effect causes moving objects and currents to be deflected to the right, while in the southern hemisphere, it causes deflection to the left.

18. D
The plasma membrane surrounds the cell and functions as an interface between the living interior of the cell and the nonliving exterior.[24]

19. B
DNA is a nucleic acid that contains the genetic instructions used in the development and functioning of all known living organisms (with the exception of RNA viruses). The DNA segments that carry this genetic information are called genes but other DNA sequences have structural purposes or are involved in regulating the use of this genetic information. Along with RNA and proteins DNA is one of the three major macromolecules that are essential for all known forms of life.[25]

20. C
Tight junctions or zonula occludens are the closely associated areas of two cells whose membranes join forming a virtually impermeable barrier to fluid. It is a type of junctional complex present only in vertebrates. The corresponding junctions that occur in invertebrates are septate junctions.[26]

21. A
The cell membrane is a biological membrane that separates the interior of all cells from the outside environment. The cell membrane is selectively permeable to ions and organic molecules and controls the movement of substances in and out of cells[27]

22. C
The plasma membrane or cell membrane protects the cell from outside forces. It consists of the lipid bilayer with embedded proteins.

23. A
Genes are made from a long molecule called DNA, which is copied and inherited across generations. DNA is made of simple units that line up in a particular order within this large molecule. The order of these units carries genetic information similar to how the order of letters on a page carries information. The language used by DNA is called the genetic code that lets organisms read the information in the genes. This information is the instructions for constructing and operating

a living organism.

24. D

A **balanced equation** is a description of a **chemical reaction** that gives the chemical formulas of the reactants and the **products** of the reaction, with coefficients introduced so that the number of each type of atom and the total charge is **unchanged** by the reaction.

Note: For example, a balanced equation for the reaction of sodium metal (Na(s)) with chlorine gas (Cl_2(g)) to form table salt (NaCl(s)) would be 2 Na(s) + Cl_2(g) = 2 NaCl(s), NOT Na(s) + Cl_2(g) = NaCl(s).[44]

25. A

Covalent bonds involve a complete sharing of electrons and occurs most commonly between atoms that have partly filled outer shells or energy levels.

Note: Diamond is strong because it involves a vast network of covalent bonds between the carbon atoms in the diamond.[28]

26. C

The reaction of elements with low electronegativity(almost empty outer shells) with elements with high electronegativity (mostly full outer shells) causes Ionic bonds.

27. D

Polar bonds involve electrons that are not equally shared, and may be deemed as an intermediate between the extremes represented by **covalent** and **ionic** bonds.

28. B

Hydrogen bonds involves an especially strong dipole-dipole force between molecules, and are responsible for the unique properties of water and pin DNA into its characteristic shape.

29. C

Henry's law predicts that the solubility (C) of a gas or volatile substance in a liquid is proportional to the partial pressure (P) of the substance over the liquid (P = k C).

30. D

Boyle's law states that the pressure of an ideal gas is inversely proportional to its volume, if the temperature and quantity of gas are held constant.

Note: Doubling gas pressure halves gas volume, if temperature and quantity of gas don't change. If the initial pressure and volume are P1 and V1 and the final pressure and volume are P2V2, then P1V1 = P2V2 at fixed temperature and gas amount.[29]

31. A

pH is a measure of effective concentration of hydrogen ions in a solution, and is approximately related to the molarity of H+ by pH = - log [H+]

32. B

Four factors that affect rates of reaction are: **Temperature, particle size, concentration, and the presence of a catalyst.**

33. A

A higher concentration of reactants causes more effective collisions per unit time, leading to an increased reaction rate.

34. B

Dalton's law is expressed by the equation: $P_{tot} = P_a + P_b$, whereby P is pressure, P_{tot} is total pressure, P_a and P_b are component pressures.

35. A

A **Metalloid** is an element with both metallic and non-metallic properties. Examples are silicon, arsenic, and germanium.

36. D

All of these statements are correct.

37. C

All the statements are false.

38. A

Brownian motion is the spontaneous, random movement of small particles suspended in liquid, caused by the unbalanced impacts of molecules on the particle.

Note: The discovery of Brownian motion provided strong circumstantial evidence for the existence of molecules.[47]

39. C

Frequency is the number of cycles of a wave that move past a fixed observation point per second.

Note: The SI unit of frequency is the Hertz (Hz).

40. D

Wavelength is the distance between adjacent peaks (or adjacent troughs) on a wave.

Note: Varying the wavelength of light changes its color; varying the wavelength of sound changes its pitch.[30]

41. D

Wavefunction is a mathematical function that gives the amplitude of a wave as a function of position (and sometimes, as a function of time and/or electron spin).
Note: Wavefunctions are used in chemistry to represent the behavior of electrons bound in atoms or molecules.[31]

42. A

The periodic table of the chemical elements (also known as the periodic table or periodic table of the elements) is a tabular display of the 118 known chemical elements organized by selected properties of their atomic structures. Elements are presented by increasing atomic number, the number of protons in an atom's atomic nucleus. [32]

43. D

In chemistry, the law of definite proportions, sometimes called Proust's Law, states that a chemical compound always contains the same proportion of elements by mass. An equivalent statement is the law of constant composition, which states that all samples of a given chemical compound have the same elemental composition. [33]

44. A

Isotopes are variants of atoms of a particular chemical element that have differing numbers of neutrons.

45. C

In chemistry and atomic physics, main group elements are elements in groups (periodic columns) whose lightest members are represented by helium, lithium, beryllium, boron, carbon, nitrogen, oxygen, and fluorine as arranged in the periodic table of the elements. Main group elements include elements (except hydrogen) in groups 1 and 2 (s-block), and groups 13 to 18 (p-block). [34]

46. A

Jacques Charles was a French chemist famous for his experiments in ballooning. Instead of hot air, he used hydrogen gas to fill balloons that could stay a float longer and travel farther.

47. D

Boyle's law (sometimes referred to as the Boyle-Mariotte law) is one of many gas laws and a special case of the ideal gas law. Boyle's law describes the inversely proportional relationship between the absolute pressure and volume of a gas, if the temperature is kept constant within a closed system. [35]

48. B

Standard temperature = 273 Kelvin

49. A

Real gases approach ideal behavior **at**

high pressure and high temperature.

50. C

Charles's Law, or the law of volumes, was found in 1678. It says that, for an ideal gas at constant pressure, the volume is directly proportional to the absolute temperature (in kelvins).[36]

Conclusion

CONGRATULATIONS! You have made it this far because you have applied yourself diligently to practicing for the exam and no doubt improved your potential score considerably! Getting into a good school is a huge step in a journey that might be challenging at times but will be many times more rewarding and fulfilling. That is why being prepared is so important.

Study then Practice and then Succeed!

Good Luck!

Register for Free Updates and More Practice Test Questions

Register your purchase at

www.test-preparation.ca/register.html for fast and convenient access to updates, errata, free test tips and more practice test questions.

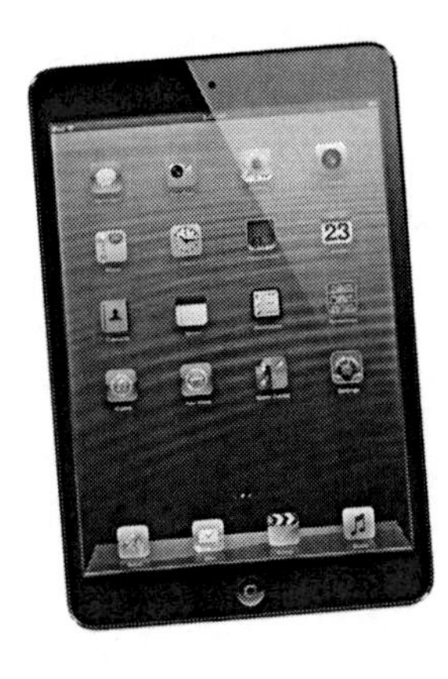

FREE Ebook Version

Download a FREE Ebook version of the publication!

Suitable for tablets, iPad, iPhone, or any smart phone.

Go to http://tinyurl.com/phagogm

DET Test Strategy!

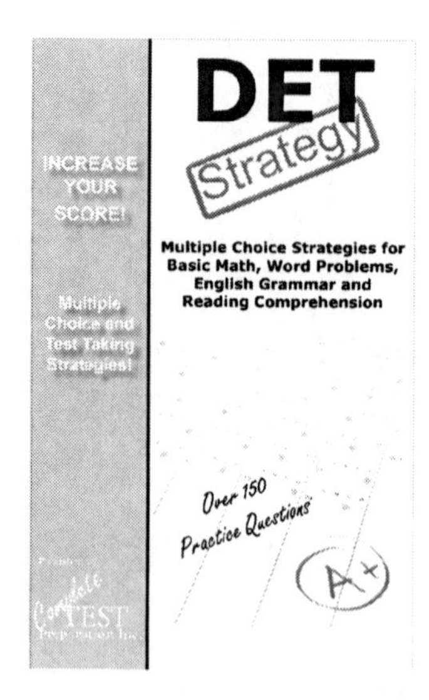

Learn to increase your score using time-tested secrets for answering multiple choice questions!

This practice book has everything you need to know about answering multiple choice questions on the DET!

You will learn 12 strategies for answering multiple choice questions and then practice each strategy with over 45 reading comprehension multiple choice questions, with extensive commentary from exam experts!

Also included are strategies and practice questions for basic math, plus math tips, tricks and shortcuts!

Maybe you have read this kind of thing before, and maybe feel you don't need it, and you are not sure if you are going to buy this Book.

Remember though, it only a few percentage points divide the PASS from the FAIL students.

Even if our multiple choice strategies increase your score by a few percentage points, isn't that worth it?

https://www.createspace.com/4126072

Enter Code LYFZGQB5 for 25% off!

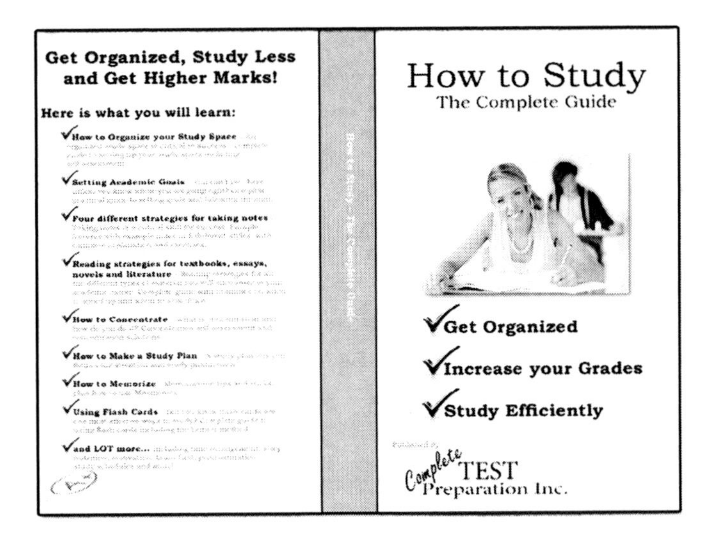
Get Organized, Study Less and Get Higher Marks!
Here is what you will learn:
How to Organize your Study Space
Setting Academic Goals
Four different strategies for taking notes
Reading strategies for textbooks, essays, novels and literature
How to Concentrate
How to Make a Study Plan
How to Memorize
Using Flash Cards
and LOT more...
How to Study
The Complete Guide
Get Organized
Increase your Grades
Study Efficiently
Complete TEST Preparation Inc.

Thanks!

If you enjoyed this book and would like to order additional copies for yourself or for friends, please check with your local bookstore, favourite online bookseller or visit www.test-preparation.ca and place your order directly with the publisher.

Feedback to the publisher may be sent by email to feedback@test-preparation.ca

NOTES

[1] Immune System. In *Wikipedia*. Retrieved November 12, 2010 from, en.wikipedia.org/wiki/Immune_system.
[2] White Blood Cell. In Wikipedia. Retrieved November 12, 2010 from en.wikipedia.org/wiki/White_blood_cell.

[3] Herr, N. (2008). The Sourcebook for Teaching Science: Strategies, Activities, and Instructional Resources. San Francisco, CA: John Wiley & Sons, Inc.
[4] Brimblecombe, S., Gallannaugh, D., & Thompson, C. (1998). QPB Science Encyclopedia: An A to Z Guide to Everything You Need to Know About Science. New York, NY: Helicon Publishing Group Ltd.
[5] Biology. In Wikipedia. Retrieved May 10, 2012 from http://en.wikipedia.org/wiki/Biology.
[6] http://upload.wikimedia.org/wikipedia/commons/a/ac/NIEHScell.jpg
[7] Classification. In Wikipedia. Retrieved January 20, 2013 from http://en.wikipedia.org/wiki/Biological_classification
[8] http://en.wikipedia.org/wiki/File:TrophicWeb.jpg
[9] Chemistry. In Wikipedia. Retrieved May 10, 2012 from http://en.wikipedia.org/wiki/Chemistry.
[10] Infectious Disease. In *Wikipedia*. Retrieved November 12, 2010 from en.wikipedia.org/wiki/Infectious_disease.
[11] Thunderstorm. In *Wikipedia*. Retrieved November 12, 2010 from en.wikipedia.org/wiki/Thunderstorm.
[12] Meteorology. In *Wikipedia*. Retrieved November 12, 2010 from en.wikipedia.org/wiki/Outline_of_meteorology.
[13] U.S. Navy Seal. In *Wikipedia*. Retrieved November 12, 2010 from en.wikipedia.org/wiki/United_States_Navy_SEALs.
[14] Gardening. In *Wikipedia*. Retrieved January 2, 2012 from en.wikipedia.org/wiki/Gardening.
[15] The Four Fundamental Forces. (n.d.) Oracle Education Foundation. Retrieved from http://library.thinkquest.org/27930/forces.htm
[16] Heat Transfer. (n.d.) HyperPhysics Online. Retrieved from hyperphysics.phy-astr.gsu.edu/hbase/thermo/heatra.html
[17] What Causes DNA Mutations? (n.d.) Learn.Genetics http://learn.genetics.utah.edu/archive/sloozeworm/mutationbg.html
[18] What is the Musculoskeletal System? (n.d).Wisegeek.com http://www.wisegeek.com/what-is-the-musculoskeletal-system.htm
[19] Respiratory System. In *Wikipedia*. Retrieved November 12, 2010 from en.wikipedia.org/wiki/Respiratory_system.
[20] Mythology. In *Wikipedia*. Retrieved November 12, 2010 from en.wikipedia.org/wiki/

Mythology.
[21] Circulatory System. In *Wikipedia*. Retrieved November 12, 2010 from en.wikipedia.org/wiki/Circulatory_system
[22] Blood. In Wikipedia. Retrieved November 12,2010 from http://en.wikipedia.org/wiki/Blood.
[23] The Skeletal System. (n.d.). virtualmedicalcentre.com http://www.virtualmedicalcentre.com/anatomy.asp
[24] Membrane. Retrieved from http://faculty.clintoncc.suny.edu/faculty/michael.gregory/files/bio%20101/bio%20101%20lectures/membranes/membrane.htm
[25] DNA. In *Wikipedia*. Retrieved November 12, 2010 from http://en.wikipedia.org/wiki/DNA.
[26] Tight Junction. In *Wikipedia*. Retrieved November 12, 2010 from http://en.wikipedia.org/wiki/Tight_junction.
[27] Cell Membrane. In *Wikipedia*. Retrieved November 12, 2010 from http://en.wikipedia.org/wiki/Cell_membrane.
[28] Covalent Bonds. (n.d.) In Plos Biology. Retrieved from staff.jccc.net/pdecell/chemistry/bonds.html
[29] Boyle's law. (n.d.) In General Chemistry Online! Retrieved from http://antoine.frostburg.edu/chem/senese/101/glossary/b.shtml
[30] Wavelength. (n.d.) In General Chemistry Online! Retrieved from http://antoine.frostburg.edu/chem/senese/101/glossary/b.shtml
[31] Wavefunction. (n.d.) In General Chemistry Online! Retrieved from http://antoine.frostburg.edu/chem/senese/101/glossary/b.shtml
[32] Periodic Table. In *Wikipedia*. Retrieved November 12, 2010 from http://en.wikipedia.org/wiki/Periodic_table.
[33] Law of Constant Composition. In *Wikipedia*. Retrieved November 12, 2010 from http://en.wikipedia.org/wiki/Law_of_constant_composition.
[34] Main Group Element. In *Wikipedia*. Retrieved November 12, 2010 from http://en.wikipedia.org/wiki/Main_group_element.
[35] Boyles Law. In *Wikipedia*. Retrieved November 12, 2010 from http://en.wikipedia.org/wiki/Boyle%27s_Law.
[36] Gas Laws. In *Wikipedia*. Retrieved November 12, 2010 from http://en.wikipedia.org/wiki/Gas_laws.

CPSIA information can be obtained at www.ICGtesting.com
Printed in the USA
LVOW09s1505171115

462983LV00014B/575/P

9 781772 450491